BABY SLEEP TRAINING

How to Help New Parents to Calm and

Train Toddler for a Healthy Sleep

June Smith

TABLE OF CONTENTS

INTRODUCTION

Anyone reading this book is likely to fall into one of two categories: either you're a type-A, get-'er-done parent who tries to prevent any sleep problems by tackling them early or stopping them before they start, or you're the parent of a baby or infant and totally exhausted as your child struggles to sleep well. The book is for you, anyway!

So many families consider success to be entirely elusive, and the fact that almost every piece of information a parent reads or receives is in direct conflict with the next complicates the determination to find the right solution. Add a massive lack of sleep for parents and baby, and it's not difficult to see why sleep problems seem to escalate so quickly.

To those of you who are reading this in preparation for your new baby in the first group, I congratulate you. Understanding the principles contained in this book will help you avoid many of the long-term problems that families tend to endure in sleep. With the reasons I'm going to go into in the coming chapters, you won't be able to stop having to sleep train your kid, but it will be more easily accomplished by not only knowing what to expect, but also knowing when and how to deal effectively with problems when they eventually occur.

Believe me, for anyone who has already read a stack of books, I know there's a lot of knowledge out there, and I also know that sleep experts tend to come across as being highly authoritative, making you feel their way is the only way. I'm not here to convince you that the Baby Sleep Trainer System is the only method, and I won't even tell you it's the best way (though hundreds of customers have told me it's valid for them). I am here to reassure you that the Baby Sleep Trainer Method works for almost any child when applied consistently, and it typically solves sleep problems with the slightest amount of crying out of any common solution. For everything I ask you to do, I will make an evidence-backed case and direct you through any blip and bump that you may encounter along the road. Patience and discipline are all you need to be effective.

Do any of those describe your child?

- My kid needs to fall asleep forever.
- My baby will fall asleep only if I do one or more of the following things: breastfeed, bottle feed, pacifier, rock, carry, swing, or ride in a car.
- My kid is awake all night sometimes.
- My baby's not going to sleep quickly or takingreally short naps.
- Are you explaining this? Are these the thoughts that cross your mind?

- I wish my baby would sleep better.
- I'm not going to — I can't — let my kid sweat it out.

If so, this book was written for you. It will explain exactly what steps you should take to help your baby sleep peacefully through the night. So, open your eyelids, grab a cup of coffee, and let me explain how to help your baby sleep — so you can also get some sleep and so you can worry no more.

Poor Sleep Sucks. Kids have incredibly common problems with sleep. More than a fifth of parents will speak with their child's pediatrician about sleep problems. This is only the tip of the ice-berg because parents tend to underreport behavioral issues out of a mistaken belief that acknowledging them as parents represents failure. Another study of parents of young children said that something about their child's sleep would improve a whopping 90 percent of parents. And sleep problems are not only normal, but they can have severe consequences.

After a sleepless night, your kids may be a bit better off than you. They can always catch a short nap in the car, or in the stroller, here and there. Now, such odd sleep cycles do not carry the same benefits as a good night's sleep. Research shows that it is difficult for exhausted children to control their actions and retain infor-mation. Small children who are deprived of sleep probably won't drift off in the sandbox. You have a much greater chance of being hyperactive, competing with peers, and being obese. And they are more likely to experience sleep problems during their childhood and adolescence, probably even into adulthood (surveys of adults with insomnia indicate that sleep problems usually begin in infancy).

So here's my promise to you: When you work through the techniques outlined in this book and remain consistent in allowing your child the time and space they need to learn how to fall asleep on their own, they'll sleep through the night and take regular naps before you know it — and that's a blessing for both of you.

Please note that some sentences in this book refer to the baby using a female pronoun and qualifier. This is not to assume that the book is made for only female children. It is solely by the author's discretion to avoid using the qualifier "it" for a baby, thanks.

CHAPTER 1: BABY SLEEP TRAINING

What exactly is SLEEP training?

Sleep training is amethod of helping a baby learn to sleep through the night and stay asleep. Most babies do this with speed and ease. But many others have difficulty going down to sleep – or getting back to sleep when they wake up, and on the way, they need assistance.

How Sleep Deprivation Affects Your Child

Parents aren't the only people that suffer extreme fatigue in the family. If it's not enough incentive to take care of yourself or your family to help your child sleep better, than we hope to know the impact of fatigue on your little one.

Evidence published in *Nature Neuroscience* suggests that early brain development, learning, and memory are all helped by good sleep, while sleep disturbance was related to behavioral and emotional problems. Many sleep-deprived infants show some signs of persistent overtiredness: cranky or fussy behavior, dark circles under their eyes, or redness around their lips, or plenty of moaning or crying all day. On the other hand, some children are even miraculously tempered even when they are deprived of sleep and manage to remain cheerful and happy during the day.However, be warned that their tiredness is still taking a toll on their development which can be difficult to see.

Kids need to get the right amount of sleep for their age to progress to their full capacity biologically, mentally, and cognitively.They still do a lot of development during sleep in the first few years of life. If they fall short of what they need, children will be deprived of one of the most important foundations to be healthy. Usually, this deprivation will manifest throughout the day as decreased alertness, less physical coordination, and increased ups and downs in emotional and behavioral ways. The body, brain, and emotions of your infant are all affected. And that is not merely a temporary phenomenon. If not addressed, sleep disturbances that occur in infancy frequently extend into later adolescence and are strongly correlated with mental, behavioral, and health issues as children grow older. In a long-term study in *The Journal of Child Psychology and Psychiatry*, infants suffering from chronic sleep deprivation were much more likely to continue suffering from sleep problems when they were five-years-old and ten-years-old than children who slept well as infants.

On the other hand, a well-rested kid— one who gets good care for the sleep— is a healthy boy. A rested child will wake up happy to greet the day, maximize her brainpower to be able to process all of the stimulation around her and generate creative problem-solving, stay emotionally and behaviorally stable throughout the day, and effectively meet her physical and cognitive needs, such as mastering the art of balancing on two legs or finding the right words to express themselves. But even if you have a girl who's a beautiful, joyful baby butbeing robbed of sleep, you don't want to give her a junky night, just as you wouldn't feed her unhealthy food for dinner.

No matter how old your child is, maintaining his or her good sleep is a crucial part of supporting his or her health. We know that you would not deliberately do anything to hinder the well-being of your child. We know you only want the best for him, and also for you. That's why you owe it to your whole family to start getting the sleep youall need so badly.

How we feel when babies cry

Just as your baby is born with some automatic, built-in reflexes (like crying) you are fitted with a lot of automatic and irresistible baby feelings. Researchers proved years ago that adults are naturally attracted to an infant's face. The heart-shaped face of your baby, upturned nose, large eyes, and full forehead give you the urge to kiss and cuddle him for hours!

You also have different senses to help you know if your baby is babbling, or if he urgently needs you. The brain not only gets the message, but the body does too. That's why your baby's cries can really "get under your skin." You feel your nervous system going into "red alert" as your heart starts pounding, your blood pressure soars, your palms sweat, and your stomach tightens like a fist. Research showsthe loud scream of a baby will jolt the nervous system of a parent like an electric shock. Scientists have also demonstrated, as you might expect, that parents with other stresses–such as fatigue, isolation, marital discord, financial stress, hormonal imbalance, family or neighbor problems, or other serious strains–are particularly susceptible to feeling overwhelmed by their baby's cries.

It's not just the sound of the cries of your baby that makes you want to support him, it's the way he looks. It can penetrate your heart like an arrow to see his little fists pounding in the air and his face twist in obvious pain. You will be compelled by every caring fiber in your body to console your crying child. This strong biological instinct is exactly why standing outside the nursery door feels so wrong whilemaking your baby cry it out.

Not just parents are tuned in to the cries of an infant. Single adults and children, too, find the sound of a baby crying upsetting. Yet new parents, especially those without prior experience in infant care, find their baby's crying extremely disturbing.

Your baby's cries may even rekindle emotional trauma forgotten from your past. Youmight suddenly remember memories of previous failures or humiliations, such as someone who was cruel to you or remember people who hated you and threatened you. The weeping canmake you feel guilty for some past misdeed. This sense of helplessness is so overwhelming for some parents that it makes them turn away from the cries of their babies and neglect their needs.

Your kid, of course, does not intend to make you feel guilty or insufficient. His screams are never, never, never deceptive, cruel, rude, or negative during the first few months of life. Also, when your baby screams on and on, those feelings can bubble up inside.

When can you start sleep training?

Many experts suggest you start when your baby is between 4 and 6 months old. Babies usually start developing a regular sleep-wake cycle by about four months and reduce most of their night feedings. These are signs that they could be ready to begin sleep training. Most babies of this age are also able to sleep long stretches of the night.

Each baby is different, of course. Some may not be ready for sleep training until they're a little older. Some babies sleep seven hours or longer at an early age, while others won't work until much later. If you don't know if your baby's ready for sleep training, ask his doctor.

What are my choices for sleep-training?

There are many different ways to teach your child about safe sleeping habits. What sort of technique shouldyou try? That depends on your child's sleep plan and what you feel comfortable doing.

Although researchers continue to debate the merits of various options for sleep training, quality seems more important than the process. An analysis of 52 sleep studies using different methods published in the journal *Sleep* found that if applied consistently, almost all of the techniques were successful.

Choose a sleep training system that you can follow through with and live with. Be versatile about how you apply it, and watch your baby's reaction carefully. If he's very stubborn or you see his overall mood and actions changing for the worse, pause and wait a few weeks before trying again or choosing another method.

Many forms of sleep training follow one of these basic approaches:

The cry it out approach

Proponents of these forms of sleep training say it's okay for your child to cry when you put him to bed and leave the room, even though they aren't promoting making a baby cry forever. These methods typically suggest putting your baby in bed when he's still awake and allowing for short periods of crying punctuated by comforting (but not picking up) your child.

The most well-known cry it out technique is the one created by pediatrician Richard Ferber, founder of Children's Hospital Boston's Center for Pediatric Sleep Disorders. Ferber says babies must learn to soothe themselves if they are to fall asleep on their own and sleep through the night. Ferber believes that teaching a baby how to soothe himself may involve allowing him to cry alone for prescribed periods.

The no-tears approach

These advocates for sleep training recommend a more gradual approach – calming the baby to sleep and providing comfort as soon as the child cries.

The fading approach

Fading, also known as adult fading or camping out, falls into the mid-spectrum of sleep training. In fading, parents gradually decrease their position in bedtime by sitting near thebaby until he/she falls asleep and pushing the chair further away from the crib every night. Another diminishing strategy is to monitor your baby and reassure her every five minutes (without picking her up) until he/she falls asleep.

Other approaches

Several experts suggest slightly different approaches to these processes. Pediatrician Harvey Karp is probably the best known. His technique recommends a very basic routine that involves the so-called five S's: swaddling, side or stomach position (to relax your infant, not to sleep), shushing, running, and sucking.

What is the way of crying it out method?

People often think that this sleep training method involves leaving the babies to cry alone for as long as it takes before they fall asleep. Yet "cry it out" (CIO) simply refers to any solution to sleep training–and there are many –that says it's okay to let a baby cry for a specified time period (often a very short time) before providing comfort.

In Ferber's 1985 book *Solve Your Child's Sleep Problems* (revised and expanded in 2006), pediatrician Richard Ferber introduced one method for getting children to sleep, which has become practically synonymous with crying it out–so much so that you can hear parents call it "Ferberizing."

Ferber himself never uses the phrase "cry it out." And he's just one of several parenting experts who suggest "cry it out" Many pediatricians believe that crying is natural and cry it out approaches work well formanyfamilies.

What's the theory behind cry it out?

The hope is that if your child is accustomed to having you rock or nurse him to sleep, he will not learn to fall asleep alone. As all children and adults do as part of the natural sleep cycle, when he wakes up during the night, he will become frightened and scream for you instead of being able to go back to sleep.

In comparison, if your baby goes to sleep at bedtime, to soothe himself he can use the same technique when he wakes up at night or during a nap.

Crying is not the aim of this form of sleep training, but advocates say it's often an unavoidable side effect when your baby learns to sleep alone. We argue that the short-term pain of a few tears is far outweighed by the long-term benefits: a kid who sleeps comfortably and peacefully on his own, and parents who can count on the remainder of a good night.

Ferber's steps of cry it out method

Step 1

Put your infant in his bed when he is sleepy but still awake.

Step 2

Tell your child goodnight, and leave the room. If he is weeping as you go, let him weep for a set amount of time.

Step 3

Go back to the room for no more than a minute or two to hug your baby and comfort him. Turnoff the light, and keep your voice quiet and cool. Don't get him. Leave when he is still awakeagain, even if he is weeping.

Step 4

Stay out of the room for a little longer than the first time and follow the same routine, remaining out of the room for increasingly longer intervals, each time coming back for just a minute or two to hug him and encourage him and leave while he is still awake.

Step 5

Implement this routine until your child falls asleep when you exit the room.

Step 6

If your child wakes up later again, follow the same procedure, starting with the minimum waiting time for that night and increasing the intervals between visits slowly until you hit the limit for that night.

Step 7

Increase the amount of time between nursery visits each evening. According to Ferber, in most situations, the kid will sleep by the third or fourth night on his own–a week at most. If after many nights of trying, your kid is very stubborn, wait a few weeks and then try again.

How long should can I leave my child alone?

Ferber suggests the following interval:

- First night: depart the first time for three minutes, the second time for five minutes and the third time for 10 minutes and all other waiting periods.
- Second night: Five minutes, 10 minutes, then 12 minutes.
- Make the intervals longer each following night.

Note there is nothing special about these waiting periods. You can choose with whichever period of time you feel comfortable with.

Practical tips for parents and professionals using a cry it out approach

- Set the stage for success by creating and sticking to a bedtime routine before you try a cry it out process. For starters, a bath, a book, a lullaby, and to bed, every night at the same time. This way you know exactly what to expect from your kids. It also helps to have a consistent schedule for the day which includes naps.
- Build a solid plan to ensure that you and your partner are prepared before you start the sleep training–both emotionally and practically.

On the practical side, launching your sleep schedule is probably not a good idea if, for example, your partner is about to set off on a business trip or if your in-laws are coming for a visit.

On the emotional side, talk to your partner about the plan and make sure that you both understand how to proceed and agree. That way if you run into rough patches, you'll be able to support each other.

- Make sure to stick to it once you start your program. Parents who have been through sleep training believe that the secret is consistency. When you know that your child is just not physically or emotionally ready and you decide to put the plan on hold for some time, follow up ina few weeks. You may be tempted to give in and catch or rock him when your baby wakes you up at 2 a.m. but if you do, your hard work will be wasted and you'll have to start over from square one.

- Intend on losing some sleep. Start the method of crying it out on a night when it does not matter if you lose a little sleep. If you're working all week, for example, you might want to start on a Friday night, so you'll be able to catch up on lost sleep by the time Monday comes.

- Plan for some tough days. It can be painful to hear your baby cry, as every parent knows. Place a timer duringthe waiting periods and go to another part of the house, or put on some music, so you don't have to hear every whimper. As one parent at Baby Center says, "The first week canbe hard. Try to relax and realize that everybody in your family willsleep easier and happier when it's all over."

- Consider it a team effort. Do something fun with your partner during the waiting periods, including playing cards or listening to music. If, after a while, you find the moaning unbearable, let your partner take over so you can take a hike or a warm bath. You should give your partner a break if you're refreshed.

- Change the way your family works. If you want to use a strategy like this but find it too extreme, a more incremental solution may be used. For example, you can spread out the seven-day plan of Ferber over 14 days, through doing the wait every other night, rather than every night. Remember your primary goal is to provide a good night's rest for yourself and your kids.

- Expect rebounding. Even after you have "done" sleep training, you can expect your child to relapse from time to time, like when he gets sick or when you're traveling.

Why are some people not comfortable using crying it out?

Many parents and parenting experts condemn making a baby cry out without instantly responding. They say it could undermine the trust of the child in his parents, and thus his sense of security in the world.

In response to such concerns, Ferber says a baby who has been given lots of attention and love during the day can be left alone at night with no permanent harm sustained.

"A young child can't understand what's best for him yet, and if he doesn't get what he wants, he can scream," Ferber writes. "If he wanted to play with a sharp knife, no matter how hard he was screaming, you wouldn't give it to him and you wouldn't feel guilty or think about the psychological consequences. Poor sleep habits are also detrimental to your child and it's your job to correct them."

View of Experts

Richard Ferber, pediatrician

''It becomes more important for you to provide increasingly consistent structure when your baby is three months old and has formed a fairly predictable 24-hour routine. If you do your best to set up a reasonable and consistent daily routine and stick to it as much as possible, then your child is likely to continue to develop good habits. If, instead, you accept constant changes in the times of your child's feedings, playtime, baths, and other activities, chances are his sleep will also become erratic.''

Jodi Mindell, psychologist

''The quicker the process works, the more realistic the baby gets to sleep. He's going to fall asleep alone, and you're going to get the sleep you need... Don't wait too long though. The sooner the better. Also, the process of getting your child on a sleep schedule and sleeping through the night becomes more complicated as your baby gets older, that is, at least 5 or 6 months.''

Kim West, licensed clinical social worker

''When you change your baby's sleep pattern, you're going to have to give up middle-of-the-night crutches, known withnegative associations, that might get her back to sleep in the short run but won't stop her from waking up in an hour again. He/she could be resisting the transition. Before it gets better, the behavior may get even worse as the babyadapts to new routines, to new positive associations."

Do I need to apply a method of sleep training to my child?

Many parents often decide to try a particular method because they are tired or irritated by the sleep habits of their child and nothing seems to work that they have tried on their own. If you are happy with the way things are, count your blessings and keep on with what you are doing.

Families have different tolerances and standards. A 9-month-old who wakes up twice a night could have one set of parents pulling out their hair while another family would not have it any other way. If your family doesn't sleep well, you'll know it–and you can call your baby's doctor for help or read up on expert methods.

Here are a few things to consider:

- Many kids are naturally good sleepers, so they fall into a sleep pattern that happens to everyone before too long. Others are often fussy or wakeful, and may need more structure to help them sleep better–or more caring.
- Each child is different, even within the same family. And if your first child's sleeping methods aren't working with the next one, you might need some new ideas.
- With a second or subsequent infant, you may not be able to cry it out because a crying baby is likely to keep your older children awake.

- You don't have to strictly follow any protocol. You may consider only one element of an effective method for your child. Feel free to take whatever you can.
- The best "process" is sometimes common sense. Parents also create their own ways of getting their children into good sleeping habits. If it works, stay tuned.
- Expect your child to relapse sometimes, even after sleep training is over, like when he/she gets sick or when you're traveling.

Typical Sleep Pattern for Newborns

Newborns needa lot of sleep, typically up to 16 or 17 hours a day. But most infants, during the first few weeks of life, do not stay asleep for more than two to four hours at a time, day or night.

The outcome? Lots of sleep and a very busy-and tiring-schedule for you. As a new parent, you'll definitely be up to change, feed, and console him several times during the night.

Why newborn sleep patterns are unpredictable

Baby sleep cycles are much shorter than those of adults, and babies spend more time sleeping in rapid eye movement (REM), which is assumed to be important for the exceptional development of their brain.

All this unpredictability is a required process for your baby and it doesn't last long-although when you're sleep-deprived it may seem like a lifetime.

When your baby will start to sleep longer

At 6 to 8 weeks of age, most babies start sleeping for shorter periods during the day and longer periods at night, although most tend to wake up for nighttime feeding. You also have shorter REM sleep cycles, and long, dark, non-REM sleep periods.

Experts say that between 4 and 6 months, most babies are able to sleep through the night for a period of 8 to 12 hours. Many children sleep for a long overnight period as early as 6 weeks, but many babies do not hit the mark until they are 5 or 6 months old, and some tend to wake up into their infancy at night. If that is your target, you will help your baby get there faster by teaching him good sleeping habits from the start.

How to establish good baby sleep habits

Here are a few tips to help your infant settle down to sleep:

- Give your baby regular nap opportunities. For the first six to eight weeks, the majority of babies cannot stay up for more than two hours at a time. When you wait longer to putyour baby down, he might become overtired and have trouble falling asleep.
- Teach your child the difference between night and day. Many babies are night owls (which you may have had a hint of during pregnancy) and will be wide awake right when you want to hit the hay. You won't be able to do much about this for the first few days. But once your baby is two weeks old, you will start teaching him to differentiate between night and day.

- When he's alert and awake throughout the day, communicate and play with him as much as you can, keep the house and its space light and cheerful, and don't worry about eliminating normal daytime distractions like a television, music, or a dishwasher. Wake him up if he is prone to sleep during feedings.

Do not play with him at night when he awakes. Keep the lights and noise low, and don'tspend too much time talking to him. He will start to figure out before long that night time is for sleeping.

- Look for signs of your kid getting tired. Look out for signs that your baby is tired. Is he rubbing his head, pulling his ear, or being fussier than usual? Try to put him down to sleep if you see these or any other signs of sleepiness. Eventually you will grow a sixth sense about the everyday routines and habits of your baby and you will instinctively know when he's ready for a nap.

- Remember the child's bedtime routine. It is never too early to begin trying to follow a schedule at bedtime. It can be as simple as getting your baby to change beds, singing a lullaby, and giving him a goodnight kiss.

- If your baby is tired but awake, put him to bed. By the time he's about 6 to8 weeks old, you should start giving your baby an opportunity to fall asleep on his own. How? When he is tired but still awake, put him down. However, not everyone agrees with this approach. Many parents choose to rock or nurse their babies to sleep because they believe it's normal and natural, because they love it, and because their baby thrives and sleeps well, or simply because nothing else seems to work. Such parents expect to get up several times through the night with their baby to help him get back to sleep.

Controversies in sleep training

A central debate in sleep training is about getting the right balance between parental soothing and encouraging the baby to soothe themselves. Families who practice parenting attachment believe that the parent will take care of the baby if he or she cries, and restrict crying to the full. Nevertheless, many common forms of sleep training, such as the Ferber Method, rely on making the baby "cry it out" for a certain number of minutes, so that so-called "self-soothing" abilities are fostered rather than over-reliance on externally-provided soothing. Some have reproached the Ferber process for being inhuman. Sleep scientists, some of whom benefit from a sleep training program, research isolated variables using "treatment attempt" methodologies that leave one confused as to what participating families did, have not planned studies that look at variables of child well-being or consequences for life. Many psychologists, however, suggest that the sleep scientists fail to take into account the subtle psychological consequences of being left alone to cry it out; they conclude: "The truth is that caregivers who habitually tend to the baby's needs before the baby gets upset, and avoid crying, are more likely to have active children than the reverse.

Baby relieving methods involve jumping, jiggling, and spinning baby while sitting in a rocking chair, doing knee bends when carrying them, feeding them comfortably, using a white noise machine or device, swaddling them, skin-to-skin touch, using a bouncer or swing to move them manually, and more. Many parentsare under the belief that you should teach a baby to self-sootheandoppose the use of most or all infant calming strategies. Some parents think it's crucial to have devices like white noise machines and swings as they encourage parents to take breaks and do something other than just hold their infant.

One approach is Behavioral Infant Sleep Intervention to effectively reduce the short-to-medium-term infant sleep problems and related maternal distress. Although this randomized approach has tried and found successful, theoretical questions about long-term harm to the emotional development of children, stress management, mental health and the relationship between child and parent remain despite their effectiveness. This approach demonstrates that it does not cause long-lasting harm or benefits to infants, the child's parents, or maternal outcomes. Parents and health care professionals should feel comfortable using these approaches to reduce the population burden of issues with infant sleep and maternal depression.

CHAPTER 2: SCIENCE OF SLEEP

Vast amounts of data have come out over the last few years to support the value of sleep for a healthy body. One thing to keep in mind is that sleep patterns are very different in babies than in older kids and adults. First, let's break down what's going on at night. While a person sleeps, his brain and body go through five distinct phases, marked either by REM (rapid eye movement) sleep, or NREM (non-rapid eye movement) sleep.1 Phases 1 and 2 are light sleep, 3 and 4 are deep sleep, and five consists solely of REM sleep. REM sleep is when dreams take place, energy is returned to the brain and body, and the brain is generally active— so active that an EEG will give an awake brain equivalent amount of activity! NREM sleep is even more restorative; it's when the body restores itself and releases a host of powerful hormones, including those that control growth, muscle development, and appetite— all essential for babies growing up.

Both sleep cycles are not fully developed in the first six months of a baby's life, and researchers then differentiate between "active" and "quiet" sleep.2 Active sleep is much like REM sleep and quiet sleep isa lot like NREM sleep. Babies (like adults) can be very,

very quickly woken during active sleep, while peaceful sleep is when they seem to be sleeping through just about everything. Although adults spend only about 25% of each night in REM sleep, three children under the age of six months spend equal portions of their sleep cycles in REM and NREM sleep, lasting between thirty and fifty minutes.4 By month six, REM sleep falls to about 30% of each period.

After a calm sleep period in babies six months and younger, or after completing a full five-stage NREM / REM cycle in older babies and toddlers, children will either start another sleep cycle—or wake up. No matter how many books I read on sleep and how many blog posts I find on how-to-sleep-train, I never see this point made: an overwhelming majority of sleep-related issues, for very young children to school-age children, are related to the inability or unwillingness of a child to fall asleep unassisted. Most babies with sleep problems depend on something to fall asleep, whether it's a pacifier, rocking chair, car seat, stroller, or twirling Mom's hair, and when they end a period of REM light-sleep, they're unable to fall back into deep sleep without that same aid.

As the night progresses, children and adults alike spend more and more time in REM sleep and less and less time sleeping in NREM. This ensures that your child's REM sleep (stage 5) can take more and more time out of a given period as the morning approaches. While the average amount of each period could be 50/50 active/quiet for very young babies and 30/70 REM / NREM sleep for older babies, adolescents, and adults, more minutes are spent early in the night in deep sleep stages, and more minutes are spent in very active/light sleep stages as night turns into morning. This is why so many families find that the first part of their child's sleep is relatively uneventful, with few or no wakings, but they tend to sleep less soundly over the course of the night and fail to fall back asleep, even with help.

Finally, keep in mind that because the sleep cycles of a baby are so short, they often change throughout the night, indicating an increased number of possible nocturnal excitements during which they will seek help to get back to sleep. Since during the first few months of life, babies spend more time in light sleep than they do as older children and adults, they are easily aroused. When a baby wakes but learns how to fall asleep on their own, they can do this with minimal disruption to their own and the sleep of their parents, quickly and easily.

All of this leads to the question: When is the ideal age for starting sleep training?

Between the ages of nine and twelve weeks, nighttime development of melatonin increases substantially, five indicating that sometime around the third month of life (counting from the approximate due date of a child if they were born prematurely), their body starts to secrete melatonin daily. Since melatonin is also present in breast milk, six nursing babies often experience increased levels if they are nursed at bedtime and all night long. While the body can control day and night sleep from birth, its ability to regulate the circadian melatonin cycle occurs closer to the third month.

Developments of sleep in the first year

Infants spend most of their time in the sleeping state during the first year of life. Sleep assessment during infancy offers an opportunity to research the effect of sleep on the central nervous system (CNS) maturation, general functioning, and future development of the cognitive, psychomotor and temperament. Sleep is essential to human life, and includes both processes of physiology and behavior. Sleep is now understood as a condition that requires intense brain activity, rather than simply a resting state. The first year of life is a period of tremendous change in both the human brain and sleep development. Nevertheless, an infant undergoes multiple sleep regressions beginning at one week, which may occur regularly or fortnightly, up to the age of 8.

The relationship between the two is important, because the CNS controls the regulation of sleep and the sleep-wake cycle.

The Long-Sustained Sleep Period (LSP) is the time period a child sleeps without waking. Between the first and second months, the duration of this period increases dramatically. Between the ages of three and twenty-one months, LSP plateaus are only rising by around 30 minutes on average. In comparison, the longest self-regulated sleep cycle of a child (LSRSP) is the time in which a child can self-initiate sleep without parental interference upon waking, without sleep problems. Such self-regulation, also called self-soothing, helps the child to use those skills throughout the nocturnal cycle consistently. Over the first four months, LSRSP increases dramatically in duration, plateaus, and then gradually increases at nine months. By about six months, when waking, most infants can sleep eight hours or more uninterrupted at night, or without parental intervention.

In terms of actual numbers, an infant aged between one and three months can sleep between sixteen and eighteen hours a day in intervals that last from three to four hours. The sleep cycle stretches to about four or five hours by three months, with the overall sleep time reducing to about fourteen or fifteen hours. We also start sleeping at three months when it's dark, and wake up when it's morning. There are two separate napping time periods across four months: mid-morning and late afternoon. The longest LSP is six hours by six months, which happens during the night. There are two-three or more-hour naps, and fourteen hours of total daily sleep time.

Sleep is a predominantly biological process but it can be viewed as an action. This ensures that through practice it can be altered and controlled, and that the child can understand. During the first four months, healthy sleep patterns can be developed to lay a foundation for healthy sleep. Usually, such behaviors involve sleeping in a crib (instead of a car seat, stroller, or swing), being put down to sleep drowsy yet alert, and avoiding unpleasant sleep experiences, such as sleep breastfeeding or using a pacifier to sleep, which may be difficult to break in the future.

Each growing child is different, and within a given range, the sleep of each child is normal at different ages. Each time the baby is laid down for bed in the first few months of life and each time he or she wakes up is an opportunity for the child to learn self-initiation in sleep and fall asleep without their caregiver's undue external help. Experts say the average bedtime for a child drops from 6 pm to 8 pm, with the optimal wake-up time ranging from 6 am to 7 am. By age four, babies typically take two to three hours a day for naps, with the third nap falling by around nine months. The amount of sleep that most babies get nightly by one year of age is equivalent to that of adults.

A number of factors have been shown to be associated with sleep consolidation issues including the personality of an infant, the degree to which he/she is breastfed vs. bottle-fed, and his/her daytime behaviors and sleepiness. Co-sleeping, here described as sharing a room or bed with parents or siblings in response to an awakening, can also be detrimental to consolidating sleep. It is important to note that none of these variables have been shown specifically to cause sleep regression problems for children.

Sleep and Waking Patterns

A newborn baby is sleeping about sixteen hours a day, but at the same time for no more than a few hours at a time. He/she traverses seven awake and sleeping cycles distributed fairly equally throughout the day and night. Such periods, which range in duration from twenty minutes to five or six hours, commence with a time of REM sleep, which include multiple REM/non-REM cycles based on the length of the sleep.

Even if the baby sleeps well for a few hours, slight arousals will typically be detected. There may seem to be a rhythm to the sleep cycle in the early weeks — shorter and longer sleep and waking times are spread over every twenty-four hour period and vary from day today.

When the infant is about three months old, the daytime sleep continues in a three-nap schedule, with the mid-morning and mid-afternoon the key naps and, in general, the early evening quick nap. The infant only sleeps about thirteen hours a day by the age of three to four months, but now its sleep pattern has developed into only four to five daily and consistent cycles of sleep, with two-thirds of her sleep happening at night. By now, the differentiation between day and night should be clear and appropriate. At this age, most infants have "settled," meaning that they sleep through most of the night, at least from a late-night feeding to early-morning.

Nearly all infants are settled by six months, and the periods of continuous night-time sleep have increased for longer periods of time. Settling cycles change with each infant, of course, and nighttime wakings of your baby may diminish very slowly, or he/she may settle rapidly, as if he/she unexpectedly forgets the remaining nighttime feedings. Some babies settlequite erratically. In any case, your baby should sleep well at night at some point between three and six months. A typical six-month-old baby has a total sleep time of about twelve or thirteen hours. Usually, overnight sleep lasts between nine and a quarter hours (and as long as 11 hours if daytime naps are short) with only rare brief wakings. He/she will also take two one-to two-hour naps a day, one mid-morning and one-afternoon naps a second. (The night nap is usually dropped around this age.) The morning nap will start between 9:30 a.m. and 10:30 a.m. on most schedules, and the afternoon nap will start between 2:00 p.m. and 3:00 p.m..

Most children still sleep nearly twelve hours at a time at one year, with nine or ten of those hours occurring at night. At this point, or within a few months, most youngsters give up their morning nap. The single nap that persists generally follows lunch which happens between the hours the two naps have already been at 12:30 or 1:00 P.M. You may see other, related changes at the transition to a single-nap schedule. Since the infant now remains awake for longer stretches, both at nap time and at night, sleep can come more easily. (This is often particularly noticeable if there were problems before.) Additionally, although the second nap may have been removed, there is usually little difference in actual sleep time: either the duration of the nap or the night sleep lengthen.

Your kid should still sleep about nine to ten hours at night by age two, with a one-to two-hour nap after lunch— about 11 and a half hours in all. Probably he/she will continue her afternoon nap until at least three years of age; some children will stop by two years of age, while others will continue to nap until five years of age. The decline in the final nap is the least predictable of all the shifts in napping growth over the first five years.

Yet most kids stop napping between their third and fourth birthdays. Those who prefer to sleep longer at night may not be able to sleep during the day, maybe eleven hours. An infant who learns this cycle of sleep too early may not make it work well throughout the day. Reducing the nighttime sleep of the child to 9 or 10 hours can allow the nap to reappear.Some children continue to nap when circumstances are particularly conducive to sleep (e.g. in the car) or in daycare or preschool (where there is strong pressure to lie quietly during a prescribed period of rest) but refuse to nap at home or on weekends.

Children need less and less sleep from age three to adolescence, but the decline is smaller and much more gradual than previously thought. When children are older, they rarely sleep and slowly start sleeping less at night, dropping from about 11 hours in pre-school years to about 10 hours in pre-adolescence. The years from the age of five to twelve are the most wakeful in the life of a child. In general, children between those ages sleep well at night, and "wake well" during the day. The opportunity to sleep in the afternoon is mostly lost (including in cultures of siesta); occasional naps can indicate sickness. A child who naps most days, especially in school, may have a sleep disorder such as narcolepsy (but, as mentioned in Chapter 18, even narcoleptic children at this age may just rarely nap). Chronic sleep loss at night can cause napping, but this pattern is unusual in school-age children; rather, behavioral change during the day is the most common result of insufficient sleep.

Rapid changes occur in the child's body during the four years of puberty but the average sleep duration remains about the same. Children between the ages of fourteen and seventeen still need at least nine hours of sleep to function optimally, but few regularly get that much, at least on school nights.

Note, the requirements for sleep vary from child to family. But, if your child gets more or less sleep, one or two hours than the amount shown for her age, you should at least presume her sleep may need to be changed. I hope the remaining chapters will help you decide if he/she's having an issue and, if he/she does, identify the cause and fix it.

CHAPTER 3: LEARN BASIC SLEEP FACTS

Why Your Child Won't Sleep

First, stressing that not all sleep problems need therapy or' fixing' is crucial. Infant sleep is highly complex and not structured at all, so at this early stage what seems like a problem may well be just what the sleep of your infant looks like. I get lots of messages from worried parents that their infant, who is two weeks old, needs to be carried and will not sleep. This can be painful for the mother, but it is a very natural approach from a young person who has been kept in the womb until so recently and whose entire system is inexperienced. However, as time progresses and the child gets older and more resilient, changes and therapy will help most of the sleep problems. Getting better sleep for your child and family unit doesn't have to be about unrealistic expectations, unattended hysterical weeping sessions, or trying to drop nighttime feeding practices before a child is ready for development. It's about setting a solid framework for safe sleeping habits without affecting the well-being of your child–yeah, we're going to improve it.

Typical sleep problems from six months on may be characterized by a refusal to sleep (taking up to three hours to go to sleep at bedtime); going to sleep quickly, then waking up on multiple occasions, often 8-10 times in a two-or three-hour period; or maybe staying awake for three hours at night, waking up at four a.m., battling daytime sleep and taking short and sporadic naps. At different stages you may experience some or even all of the above. If you are, please know this is the start of the end of frustration and stress.

The structure of your child's sleep has been neurologically locked up from about six months of age and the previously disorganized essence of baby sleep is starting to become more ordered. It looks more or less like adult sleep at this point, except that the young child needs more sleep than an adult and they also dream more. Essentially, your child will start cycling through their natural phases of sleep, and this is where problems can begin to arise. Beginning to get more agitated is not uncommon for a' dream' or' textbook' baby. Likewise, you can note that at about six months, things that began at birth will get even worse. This often correlates with what is considered the'six-month relapse,' and I recommend that from this period forward it is time to really start working on sleep problems effectively. I want you to become more informed and understand why your baby doesn't sleep.

How do we sleep?

We fall asleep, we sleep all night, and then, in the morning, we wake up. Exactly right? Incorrect. We pass through a sleep cycle during the night, riding it up and down like a wave. We pass through light sleep to dream all night long into deep sleep. Between those points, we come to the surface momentarily, without fully awakening. We may be fluffing a mattress, straightening a blanket, or turning over, but we normally fade back into sleep with nary an episode memory.

Our sleep is regulated by an internal body clock that scientists called the biological clock or circadian rhythm (in Latin "about one day"). And they found that this clock is oddly set on a twenty-five-hour day— meaning we must reset it constantly. We do this with our patterns of sleep-wake, and exposure to light and darkness. Also this biological clock has specific times of the day which are programmed for sleep or awakens. That's the cause of jet lag as well as the issues of sleep that affect shift workers. That's also why it's often hard to wake up on Monday morning— sleeping in and going to bed late during the weekend upsetsroutines formed, and we have to reset our inner clocks, starting with the moment the alarm rings on Monday morning. This circadian rhythm influences how alert we feel in the course of different parts of the day. Sleeping and wakefulness are common stages. The brain seeks a state of physiological equilibrium between sleep and wakefulness, and we feel tired when the scale is high against sleep. This cycle explains why many people have a midafternoon depression, and why a siesta (afternoon nap) is regularly integrated into the day by some cultures. The human biological clock has a normal decrease in alertness in the afternoon, followed by a period of wakeful energy that lasts until later in the evening when somnolence starts. When life phases change, those patterns change. The pattern of a baby is not the same as that of an older child, the pattern of an infant is different from that of an adult, and that of an adult is different from that of an elderly person.

How do babies sleep?

An infant is not born with the circadian rhythm of an adult. The sleep-wake cycles of a newborn baby are extended all day and night, slowly settling into a rhythm of established naps and nighttime sleep.

The biological clock of a baby starts to develop at about the age of six to nine weeks and does not function smoothly until about four or five months. A baby reaches a point as the developmental process matures when he/she is mostly awake during the day and mostly asleep during the night. By about nine to ten months, the sleep periods of a baby are shortened so that every day he/she gets up and goes to sleep at about the same hours, so her stretches of sleep are longer. Because the biological clock is the main control of the rhythms of everyday sleep and wakefulness, it is easy to see why a baby doesn't sleep through the night — and why this trend affects new parents so badly! Babies are going through the same stages of sleep as adults but their periods are shorter and more frequent. Interestingly, babies spend much more time in light sleep than adults do, and they have a lot more of those brief waking periods in between. There are two reasons an infant should sleep like a baby. The first is evolutionary. The rhythm of a baby's sleep promotes brain growth and physical growth. In the first two years of life, babies grow at an astronomical rate, and their sleep patterns represent biological needs that differ greatly from adults'. The second reason a baby sleeps like a baby is because of protection. A majority of the time they spend in lighter sleep. This is most likely so that in unpleasant or threatening situations they will quickly awaken: hunger, wetness, discomfort or pain. Yes, in *The Baby Book* (Little, Brown and Company, 1993), acclaimed pediatrician Dr. William Sears says, "Encouraging a baby to sleep too deeply, too early, may not be in the baby's best interest in survival or development." Both stages of sleep are vital for the growth and development of your baby. When he matures, so does his sleep cycle; it is a biological process to achieve sleep maturity.

A baby's sleep cycle

Learning that a baby follows a specific sleep cycle naturally and inevitably is critical to understanding her struggles with falling asleep and staying that way. A typical baby's sleep cycle at night looks like this:

- Drowsy
- Falling asleep
- Light sleep
- Deep sleep for about an hour
- Brief awakening
- Deep sleep for about one to two hours
- Light sleep
- Brief awakening

- ➢ Rapid eye movement (REM)
- ➢ Dreaming sleep,
- ➢ Brief awakening
- ➢ Light sleep
- ➢ Brief awakening
- ➢ REM (dreaming sleep)
- ➢ Brief awakening
- ➢ Toward morning; another period of deep sleep
- ➢ Brief awakening
- ➢ REM (dreaming sleep)
- ➢ Brief awakening
- ➢ Light sleep
- ➢ Awake for the day

What Is a Sleep Problem?

An infant wakes up regularly during the night during the first year of life. This is not a concern, as you have learned now. It's just a biological fact. The question is our understanding of how a baby will sleep, and our own desire for an uninterrupted sleep night. We parents want our long stretches of sleep to perform our best in our busy lives, and need it. The intention then is to gradually, politely, and deliberately change the behavior of our baby to align more closely with our own needs.

How much sleep do babies need?

All babies are different, and some really need less (or more) sleep than shown here, but the vast majority of babies have similar needs for sleep. If your baby doesn't get close to the amount of sleep on this map, he may be overtired chronically— and this will affect the quality and duration of both his nap and night sleep. Your baby may not seem exhausted, but overtired babies (and kids) don't always act — at least not in the manner we expect. They may instead be clingy, hyperactive, whiny, or fussy. We may also avoid sleep, failing to understand that sleep really is what they need.

What About Nighttime Feedings

We've also heard of those three-month-old babies who sleep ten to twelve straight hours each night, without waking up for feeding. It's a mystery why these babies sleep so healthily. But when we learn about these incredible babies, we believe that all babies can and should do that, and we become very disheartened when our five-month-old, eight-month-old, or twelve-month-old wakes up for feeding twice a night. To my shock, sleep specialists— even the hardest cry-it-out advocates— agree that some children are really hungry after about four hours of sleep until they are twelve months old. If your child wakes up hungry, they suggest that you respond promptly by feeding her.

Experts also accept that a baby does not only want to grow and thrive but may also require feedings for one or two times per night for up to around nine months of age. Of course, it can be hard to know if your baby is hungry, or if she'sjust searching for warmth with breastfeeding or a bottle. When you follow the steps in this book, your baby will start to wake up less often just for warmth and your company, and when he wakes up because he's hungry, it will become more noticeable. As a baby's diet matures, she will be able to go without feeding for longer periods at night. This phase is a biological one. Research shows that feeding a good baby food at night does not help her sleep longer— although some moms swear it makes a difference with their children. You should play with that if your doctor gives you the go-ahead to feed your baby solids. But don't rush it. Babies who start solids too early tend to develop more allergies to food so it's not wise to start too early.

So it's fair that if your baby has slept for about four hours, wakes up and looks hungry you would consider feeding him. (This is particularly important if your baby is younger than four months.) Maybe he'll sleep another four hours instead of constantly waking up from hunger! Many babies also go through growth spurts where they eat more during the day and they may also sleep more at night.

What Are Realistic Expectations?

Some babies awaken up to six months two or three times a night, and up to one year once or twice a night; others awaken from one to two-years-old once a night. A baby is deemed to sleep through the night when he/she sleeps five consecutive hours, usually from midnight until 5:00 a.m. While this may not be your idea of a night's sleep, it is the fair yardstick by which we calculate the sleep of a child. That's five hours— not the 8, 10, or 12 hours we might want! The challenging part of this is that if you put your baby down at 7:00 p.m. to sleep, you're only going to catch up with your daily tasks. Just about the time you're going to bed, your baby's been sleeping for four or five hours and maybe ready for your attention. The good news is that if your baby is biologically ready, you can promote progress towards that 5-hour milestone; once your baby has achieved it, you can take steps to lengthen this stretch of time.

What Is the Right Way to Teach a Baby to Sleep?

There have been no scientific experiments on how best to teach a child to sleep but I can make a few conjectures. I doubt it's possible to enforce a regular pattern of sleeping and being awake on babies immediately after birth or that anyone should even try. We seem to need to mature their biological clocks before they can keep track of the time of day. But the same types of hints that work for us will work on the clocks of children as they develop. When you understand how much sleep your child needs, setting a daily routine and sticking with it is the most important strategy for optimizing his or her sleep. Between the ages of five months and five years, the social signals imposed by the parents become the primary factor in sleep patterns for children.

CHAPTER 4: BEDROOM ENVIRONMENT

Before you get into the strategies that will help your child get the sleep sheneeds as soon as possible — with as few cries as possible — let's address the value of a good sleep setting.

One common mistake parents make is to not ensure that they have their child's bedroom ready beforethey begin sleep training. Implementing such basic guidelines can even help to achieve better quality birthday sleep. While it is not a magic bullet to fix night waking and short naps, ensuring a sleep-conducting atmosphere will guarantee that their sleep will last longer and be of greater, more restorative quality until your child learns to fall asleep unassisted.

Next, make sure the baby's room is as dark as possible, not only at night but also early in the morning and during naps. Light, especially sunlight, has more effect on our circadian rhythms than any other signal that the body uses to control its internal clock. Sunlight interacts with photosensitive ganglion cells inside the retina, sending a message to the brain that it's time to wake up and begin the day. Particularly in the early hours of the morning, when the baby spends so much of each sleep cycle in light stage sleep, the last thing parents want is to come in at 5:30 a.m to wake them up (especially when they may have slept for another one or two hours if the room was darker).

Darkness also helps the body get more restorative, longer lasting sleep, during naps. Don't worry, keeping the nursery dark during naps won't cause the baby to have day/night confusion, which usually fixes itself in the first few weeks of a baby's life by itself. Parents will try to close all windows and switch off or cover any artificial light sources (such as little lights on TVs or fans). When light streams through the drape's edges, try sticking Velcro to the wall and curtain to cover it as tightly as possible. Make sure the hallway light is off when entering the room to check on or attend baby, so as not to add bright light. A good rule of thumb is that the room should be dark enough that you can'tread the words clearly on this post, even at noon. Try using a lamp with a fifteen-watt light bulb at night, switched on during feedings or change of diaper only if necessary. Red light has the fewest negative effects on sleep, so the best choice for nighttime tasks is a dim red lamp.

Second, during all naps and throughout the night, use true white noise, avoiding stuffed animals that turn off after a certain amount of time and any noise that has audible beats or loops. A white noise machine generating a steady fan-like sound, or just using a noisy fan facing the wall, can help baby sleep more easily and stay asleep longer. Even during sleep, and especially when going between sleep cycles (when sleep is very, very light), our brains keep processing sounds. Ambient noises will bring us out of sleep and into the wakeful state altogether. White noise needs the vigilance of the brain but does not cause it to wake up, allowing it to block out any disturbing noises. When woken by a loud sound, an adult can usually put herself back to sleep very quickly, but babies are often resistant to going back to sleep, especially in the early morning. Finally, white noise has been shown to minimize brain wave amplitude, causing the brain to fall faster into longer periods of deep sleep.

Third, video displays are a must. It will become apparent in the coming chapters why it is important to be able to monitor your child's specific sleeping and waking moments to get through sleep training as painlessly as possible. Additionally, video cameras can help identify potential hazards without having to be in the baby's room at all times. An infant or kid, for example, can pull up the mattress sheet and get stuck in it. If parents cannot track their baby visually at all times, they should not conduct any sort of sleep training whatsoever. Parents should also make sure they do not make the common mistake of putting a video camera (or, for that matter, a white noise machine) in or on the crib. Some families put a camera on the crib ledge to allow them to get a clear view, but anything on a crib can fall and injure the infant. Cameras should be mounted on the wall or put away from the crib on furniture, while ensuring that no wires or cords are within the baby's reach. When babies grow older, so does their dexterity and reach, so cameras and other objects should be kept out of sight.

Eventually, a secure portable crib or playpen-style (PPS) crib is necessary for babies before they reach an age where they start trying to climb out, usually about eighteen months, up to four years of age. A crib or PPS should have a perfectly flat mattress with no inclinations or heights. To relieve reflux symptoms, many parents are advised to lift one end of the crib or mattress, but this can very easily cause a baby to roll down to the other end and get stuck, even with very minor inclinations. The snugly fitting mattress, a very closely wrapped blanket, and the baby should be inside the crib. A mesh bumper, a single lovey twelve inches square or smaller, and a pacifier are the only other suitable products. (Note that pacies are only good if a baby can quickly put it back in his mouth on hisown, and you must first get pediatric permission to put your baby to sleep with a pacifier in the first twelve months of life.)

No other toys, covers, bumpers, pillows, rice inside tube socks, and particularly no inserts or sleeping positions should be inside the crib. If a parent feels that a baby needs a blanket, they should use a portable sleep sack instead. Any child under the age of twelve months with pillows or fluffy bumpers inside the crib has zero protection, and if a child bumps their head into crib slats, parents can buy individual crib slat covers, or have baby sleep in a mesh-sided playpen. Mobile phones are not technically off-limits, but often offer babies little benefit after a few months, and can be a hassle for older babies trying to fall asleep. Such four elements of darkness, white noise, a monitoring system, and a protected crib are all important for babies to experience healthy sleep in their childhood and infancy.

Perfect temperature for your baby

The perfect 68-72F (20-22.2c) temperature is a comfortable bet for keeping your baby cozy. Babies aren't as adaptable to temperature change as adults, according to Children's Hospital of Philadelphia. Use your own gut check to decide if your baby is not too hot or not too cold, but do not hesitate to take advice:

Signs your baby's room is too cold

- Hands or nose may be cool to the touch, but make sure there is no freezing in the heart (chest area).
- Lookout for blue lips. If your baby's room is too cold, go ahead and add one more layer under her pajamas, like a onesie.

SIGNS The BABY'S ROOM IS TOO HOT

- Sweating
- Dampness
- Quick heart rate

Always be careful and don't let the foolish deeds take hold of common sense. Do not use a space heater (especially not around window coverings) in your baby's room.

A sleep-friendly environment

Though sleeping through the night is not going to come for quite some time and every baby is special, try to make her room sleep-friendly at night from early on. Please take your baby up at bedtime, even if it's late at the start. Ensure the room is sleep-inducing, with blinds or curtains blocked out. Provide dim light for your bedtime feed and pre-sleep ritual. Switch off the lamp when it's sleep time and remove hall lighting and bathroom lamps; use only the room's 4W night light, or use the baby monitor display. Perform nocturnal feeds in the dark (use night light if it is too bright or poor lamplight) and non-stimulating. Most psychologists suggest you avoid talking to your baby or staring at it, but I am not supporting this strategy. Practice childcare at night but don't over-stimulate. Be realistic–nocturnal feed should be short, and the faster everyone gets back to sleep the better. Exclusively keep the night feeds in the bedroom–adjusting the place will generate changes of time, and can wake up your baby entirely. Once you are confident, change the nappy overnight only when you feel it is necessary and if it is, do so mid-feed, so that in the second part of the feed they can get sleepy.

CHAPTER 5: NEWBORN SLEEP

In 1992, the American Academy of Pediatrics issued its recommendation that children sleep on their backs only from birth to twelve months, greatly reducing the number of infant deaths known as SIDS (Sudden Infant Death Syndrome). That middle-of-the-night and life-saving advice, though, had an unexpected side effect: now, baby needs help falling asleep. Previously, parents were generally advised to put baby to sleep on their stomach, which usually results in newborns running less often, getting longer periods of uninterrupted sleep, and going back to sleep with less aid. Let's be clear, a newborn may sleep on her stomach more easily, but through the twelfth month of life all babies should always be put to sleep on their backs. No amount of sleep is worth the very real chance of stomach sleep suffocation.

As almost all babies are now put to sleep on their backs, parents quickly find that they have to help them fall asleep for naps and at bedtime, throughout the night, and sometimes in the middle of a nap. Techniques could include a close swaddle, a specially designed sleep rocker, and co-sleeping, all of which will be addressed in this chapter in more detail. Since it is entirely appropriate for newborn babies to develop dependency on some form of assistance to fall asleep (just as it is developmentally appropriate for young children to use training wheels on their bicycles), parents should not waste any time trying to avoid "bad habits."

It should also be remembered that some newborns will sleep up to eighteen to twenty hours a day for what might seem like an incredibly long time! Some newborn sleep is REM sleep (during which dreaming takes place), and their sleep cycles will become more normal as they develop. As an infant reaches four months and their sleep cycles become more and more like adults, parents frequently find an upswing in nocturnal arousal and an increased difficulty in getting them to sleep again. The older a baby is, and the more aware they become, the more likely they are to struggle to fall asleep and need more support, whether through rocking, feeding, etc.

So, what can you do to help your newborn not only get the sleep they need but also lay a strong foundation for future sleep?

1. Take a look at how the newborn likes to sleep. In general, swaddling is considered safe as long as they are not able to flip over, although you should also consult with your pediatrician to make sure they recommend it to your infant. It is wise to try to stop focusing on feeding as you know how your baby likes to be soothed (whether it's bouncing on a yoga ball, being brought into a dark room with loud white noise for a break from any commotion, or hanging out in a swing or bouncer that's moving

quickly). Of course, holding your baby awake while feeding will be next to impossible in the early weeks; but, as time goes by, helping them fall asleep in other ways will be easier and easier. Feeding-to-sleep can be difficult to get rid of, but stopping it from the outset is often safer. If your child is sleeping anywhere other than an empty crib, please note that they should always be within your direct line of sight. A baby of any age should not, under any condition, be allowed to sleep unsupervised in anything other than an empty crib.

2. Make sure that as they move past the sixth week of life (when newborns tend to spontaneously rise from sleep and are not as likely to fall asleep anywhere and everywhere as they used to), you start putting them to sleep in a very dark room with constant white noise for both naps and at night. The white noise system will make a continuous whirring sound— imitatingocean, rain, and lullabies sounds. If you consider noise, note that babies are exposed to constant sound in the womb, as loud as a lawnmower! Make it safe for your baby's ears as long as the white noise machine isn't deafening.

3. The American Academy of Pediatrics suggests sharing rooms (but not sharing beds) from birth through at least the sixth month of life, but preferably the twelfth. If you feel like placing your newborn in their own space, consult with your health care provider first.

4. Ensure health is your utmost concern wherever baby sleeps. Cribs should be completely flat, without any inside

bumpers, pillows, blankets, or any other items. Small movies are technically safe, less than twelve inches long, but are inappropriate for newborns. Likewise, mesh bumpers are considered safe in the first weeks of life but are unnecessary. Sleep-sack-style woven blankets are a great idea if your child might be cold at bedtime and a parent is concerned.

5. If a baby takes naps or sleeps away from his parent or caregiver at night, a video monitor should be on them at all times, and they should only sleep in a room other than their parent's direct pediatric-approved bedroom.

Where your newborn baby sleeps is as critical as how they sleep. The safest place in your bedroom is a flat, empty crib, or portable Pack-n'-Play-style crib. Also a safe option when used as directed are side-car-style baby sleepers that pull right up to the side of parents' bed. Although many parents find that their babies sleep well in co-sleepers, swings, "nests" to be used in tents, bassinets, and rockers, the general consensus is that these are not secure when used without direct supervision; however, parents can find that their pediatrician allows their use in many circumstances.

Parents may assume that elevating the crib mattress to alleviate reflex symptoms is healthy, but that is not the case, nor are there any kinds of sleep positions or wedges in a crib. In fact, no matter how safe the crib may be, every new parent may testify that all babies end up sleeping in many other locations. Make sure if your baby sleeps in a stroller, car seat, chair, or bouncer, swaddled or not, they're always in sight and earshot. Each year babies die from as-phyxiation when their chins tuck too tightly from a seated position in their car seat to their chest. The same applies to any form of cover or carrier— always be careful to make sure that your baby can breathe easily. Finally stop, as simple and tempting as it might be, to sleep on a couch or chair with your child. Especially when you are deprived of sleep, it is vital that every care is taken to ensure that the baby is never in an unsafe position at a time when you may fall asleep so deeply that you will not notice.

Early Newborn Stage: Birth through Week Six

Parents will find during this timethat their babies mostly sleep everywhere, particularly while on the go or in detention. In rare cases, very young newborns will weep fitfully, and this is usually a sign of either intestinal discomfort or a question of feeding, like not having enough breast milk yet. Any extreme crying during this periodshould be brought to your pediatrician's attention.

Within the first six weeks, moms will focus on developing the feeding relationship, whether through breastfeeding or bottle/for-mula. Mum will concentrate on rest and loving her new son. If any feeding problems arise, particularly for mothers who breast-feed, they should be addressed immediately with the aid of a lac-tation consultant. While a few common sleep books recommend some sort of sleep training beginning within the first twelve weeks of life, outcomes are inconsistent, and the stress is not worth an unpredictable outcome for both the parents and child.

If parents are involved, they may start adopting practices like swaddling, white noise, and using a pacifier to help soothe their fussy baby. Families should ensure that their baby sleeps at a single stretch from about 7:00 a.m. for more than two hours, if possible. Till 9:00 p.m.— anything after that can be considered sleeping at night. After waking the baby from a long nap, try to keep them awake (including feeding time) for thirty to fifty minutes, and then sleep again. Limiting the lengths of naps in the early days and weeks to no more than two hours is the single best thing parents can do to rapidly overcome day/night uncertainty and allow baby to have longer periods of overnight sleep.

Late Newborn Stage: Week Six through Week 16

That can be an especially challenging moment. It's usually about week six when babies get much more alert, and reflex problems frequently come up. Your previously calm and peaceful baby may now become fussy, even inconsolable, particularly around dinnertime — the newborn witching hour.

It is around this age that parents will try to establish healthy sleep patterns in earnest. The room should be very quiet, with loud white noise every time the baby sleeps at home. If co-sleeping is a strong preference, parents should try to make a priority for sleeping in a crib, Pack' n Play, or side-car co-sleeper, making sure that the baby is swaddled snugly (until the baby can turn over; then swaddling will stop immediately).

Every day, parents will start to set a "peak" time to wake baby up. This willprobably be more or less the same time every morning, but it can differ by around thirty to sixty minutes. No matter when the baby wakes, parents will start instilling a routine of sleeping, staying awake, and falling asleep. This process may be developed at the Early Newborn Stage, but it will be easier to do after week six once the baby is slightly more awake and conscious. Since setting a starting time for each day and ensuring that the baby does not sleep for any single nap for more than two hours, the most important thing parents should concentrate on is to ensure that the baby stays as awake as possible during the feeding time. At first, try one feeding each day for a baby that is used to eating and sleeping at the same time, during which the baby is fed immediately upon waking. Parents can help baby stay awake by undressing her, rubbing a cool washcloth over herface, or halfway through feeding, and changing herdiaper. Even if the baby sleeps or dusts, they should be woken soon after the feeding is over and kept awake until a sleeping signal is shown. This wakeful period can last from thirty to ninety minutes, depending on the time of day and the baby. Then baby should be assisted in falling asleep in any way that does not (if possible) require feeding.

Generally speaking, newborns have shorter times early in the day when they are comfortably awake before they need to sleep, and increase their cycles of happily waking towards the end of the day. In order to recognize the sleep signs of their baby (bearing in mind that a small percentage of babies seem to show no signs of sleep at all), parents will begin to watch baby closely thirty to forty minutes after waking. Typical signs that a baby is ready to sleep include eye rubbing, fussiness, abrupt disengagement, yawning or staring at whatever they were doing. Sleep signs can vary widely but after careful observation, most parents can learn to recognize them.

As soon as a sleep warning is heard, a parent will swaddle the baby immediately and take them to a dark room with loud white noise, if possible. Anything but feeding should be used at this stage to try and help baby sleep. Some great strategies are rolling, swaying, shushing, sitting on a yoga ball, using a pacifier etc. Baby can also sleep in a swing or rocker, with clear one-on-one monitoring (and pediatric approval). She should be fed after a baby falls asleep and wakes again, even though their last feeding was less than two hours in advance. The suggestion that an infant should only be fed every three to four hours during the day for the purpose of extending night sleep usually does not result in prolonged night sleep. Rather, it is actually the daily process of feeding, being awake, sleeping, and eating again that allows the body to sleep over longer nightly periods. Establishing this process means that babies have regular chances of feeding throughout the day and facilitates fewer night wakings. Formula-fed babies may not be ready to eat right after waking, particularly after a short nap, so after about fifteen to thirty minutes parents may wait and try feeding again, ensuring that baby stays awake the entire feeding.

Contrary to popular belief, the standard of nighttime sleep does not require an elaborate bedtime routine. In reality, all that babies need to know to understand sleep times is a brief routine. Families should feed a baby in a well-lit room about half an hour before bedtime (which may be as late as 11:00 p.m. for newborns or as early as 6:00 p.m. for a three-month-old).Ensure that the baby is kept as fully awake as possible, and then continue with pajamas and swaddling, or a bath. Darkness, white noise, and the baby's own body will be the best triggers for getting the baby to know it's time to go to bed.

As we have learned, what happens in the daytime has a direct impact on how well a newborn sleeps in the evening. Nevertheless, other evening activities can also enable the baby to sleep overnight more soundly. Parents should stop changing their baby's diaper and/or unswaddling them from bedtime (whatever parents find it to be) until morning, unless it is absolutely necessary. When changing a diaper, it should be done either whengoing from one breast to the next or halfway through a baby finishing a bottle. Parents should also make sure they use low lighting (fifteen watts and under) or no lighting at night.

The 5 "S's": Five Steps to Turn on Your Baby's Calming Reflex

Traditionally, parents and grandparents have used five distinct womb-like characteristics to soothe their children. I am referring to those time-honored "calm components" as the 5 "S's":

1. Swaddling-tight wrap
2. Side / Stomach— on her side or stomach
3. Three laying a baby. Shushing— loud white sound
4. Swinging— rhythmic, jiggly

5. Sucking— sucking onto a pacifier on anything from your nipple or finger

These five techniques are extremely effective, but only when done exactly correctly.

CHAPTER 6: GENTLE SLEEP-SHAPING APPROACH: BIRTH TO SIX MONTHS

Some parents may find it extremely challenging when your new arrival doesn't seem to be' sleeping like a baby.' New babies require a lot of sleep–around 12–16 hours a day– but this is rarely the case in large segments of time, and they don't value your night sleep! Usually, their need for sleep is met over a 24-hour period, eating every 1–3 hours and for varying durations sleeping every 1–2 hours.Childhood sleep is probably the biggest difficulty faced by parents with a relatively healthy child and it is not shocking that reports regularly indicate that 30–60% of all households have a possible sleep problem based on which re-search you read.

You may be alarmed as a new parent to discover that sleep does not come naturally to your little baby and that you, in this de-partment, need considerable assistance.Beautiful pictures of sleeping infants and well-rested new mums can be the opposite of the reality of becoming a parent and trying to get a handle on all the needs of your baby–feeding, winding, bathing, dressing and, of course, making sure they (and you) are well-rested.

Others may need extra help with what comes naturally to some children; and that isn't a knock on you as a parent, it's more to do with the personality of your child and your experience. I still come across parents telling me they think they've struggled. I inform them right away that this is not going to be the case. There are many variations in what babies can do and it's not straightforward. You can be proactive, however, and work towards better sleep without getting crazy. Whatever the temperament of your new baby–from easy to less easy–they all need considerable amounts of sleep within the first year, so don't be fooled into thinking that perhaps your baby needs less than all the others just because they always seem to be fighting to go to sleep.

Also, don't panic if your baby isn't a' good' sleeper; you can program all babies to sleep better in time. Be patient and rational–plan to get exhausted when you start on your new parenting work, whether it's your first time or you've already had kids. It's a full-time, full-on job and is different for every kid. For others what works may not work. Just be respectful to yourself and your baby; every night is a task underway.

I don't really believe a standardized sleep learning program is appropriate for young infants, particularly not before six months and probably even later, depending on the problems.

That said, I am a firm believer in helping families develop good sleeping habits in the early months, if at all necessary–without putting anybody under undue pressure. For your baby, this is a very different time, with sleep biologically disorganized and their patterns predominantly governed by the need to eat when hungry and sleep in between. That said, it's also a blank landscape where you can begin to sleep better as soon as your child can. Here are some ideas on how to do this, but we'll look first at guidelines for safe sleep.

Safe sleep to reduce the risk of SIDS

Please put your baby to sleep on their back.

- Babies lying on their tummies have a higher risk of death by cot.
- Placing your child alongside youis not healthy.
- When the baby is older and ready to roll back and forth, let them choose their own sleeping position, having previously put them on their back at the beginning of their nap.

Before and after birth, keep your baby smoke-free.

- Smoking dramatically increases the risk of death from cot.
- Don't let anyone smoke in a car or at home.
- If an adult smokesyou should not share your baby's bed with them.

Think carefully about sharing beds based on recommendations. Bed-sharing may also increase the risk of suffocation or clogging. If:

- either parent smokes(even if not at home)

- either parent has taken alcohol, narcotics or medicine, or you are extremely tired, don't share a bed with baby.

Or if the infant:

- was born prematurely (before 37 weeks), or
- had a low birth weight (less than 2.5 kg or 5.5 lbs).

The cot in your bedroom is the safest place for an infant to sleep for at least six months.

- Place the infant on the foot of the cot, so that they can't get under the blankets.
- Tuck protects the back of the infant lightly and tightly, but not deeper, which guarantees that they can not fall over the top of the baby.
- Make sure the head of your child remains uncovered.
- Keep your cot free of loose and fluffy bedding, furniture, bumpers, duvets, etc.
- Use a new, sturdy, and stable cot mattress that fits your cot properly. For everybody, the mattress should be fresh.

Don't let the baby get too hot.

- A baby that is overheated has an increased risk of death by cot.
- Don't wrap your child in too many covers.
- Best cotton cell blankets.
- Do not use duvets, pillows, or quilts.
- Baby is not allowed to wear a hat.

- Bestambient temperatures vary from 16–20 ° C (62–68F).
- Never put your cot in the proximity of a fan, heater, or fire or in direct sunlight.

When possible, breastfeed your infant.

- Breastfeeding lowers the risk of death by cot.
- Keepbreastfeeding as long as possible.

Consider a maniac.

- Some studies suggest that each time your baby goes to sleep using a dummy reduces the risk of death by cot.
- If you use a dummy instead sell it at any time of night.
- If you breastfeed, postpone the start for one month until the feeding has been identified.
- Don't worry when the dummy is falling asleep.
- If your infant is stubborn, don't push the plug.
- Do not add wires or cables to dummy.
- Never dip your dummy into chocolate, butter, honey, or other food or beverage.

Provide monitored tummy time. Allow them to spend some time on their tummy while the baby is up, and sit up while you are supervising.

- Recommended from birth.
- Please put baby on a flat, firm surface.
- Ideally, do this for 3–5 minutes, three days a day, then build up gradually for longer sessions.

Routine sleep in the house is not recommended for car seats, chairs, baby seats, and similar devices. Don'tfall asleep on the couch or armchair with your baby, as the risk increases significantly.

- Sleeping isitting up will cause breathing problems.
- Once you are done, take your baby back to sleep as soon as possible.
- Babies should not be left unsupervised for long periods of time in a seated position.

If your kid feels unwell, get early and fast medical advice.

A flexible feeding and sleeping rhythm

Ideally, the early days and weeks should be spent getting to know each other, learning about your new role and helping your kid grow to feel loved by caring for every need they have. Although most parents don't want a strict routine, and I would understand, if you have some consistency to your day and your nights, it can be very beneficial.

A regular 7 a.m. wake-up time And 7:30 hrs. It is a good beginning. This will help to stabilize your first feeding and control the daytime sleep clock in your body. Bedtime can actually start very late, but you can monitor the time that you all wake to start the day.

Learning to read your baby's sleep language

It is important that you get to know each other. It's extra important to recognize your baby's sleep signals. Having a regular daytime schedule will allow new parents to read the baby's food and sleep signs right, and everything in between. Understanding what your baby cando when you start getting tired can also be the next positive step in proper sleep hygiene.

The ' tired ' signs – the ones you will know and respond to – are:

1. A brief yawn
2. A brief zoning out or snuggling in
3. Decreased activity
4. A brief rubbing of the eye

Such signs indicate sleep preparation, and most infants will be able to go to sleep relatively easily, given the opportunity.

Signals of late sleep may be represented by:

1. Intense eye rubbing
2. Wide yawning
3. Increased activity–clenching fists/arching back
4. Agitation
5. Noise–whining/moaning/crying.

Any or all of the above indicates the over-tiredness of your baby. This may mean they'renot going to try to go to sleep, even if they're very exhausted. You have skipped their optimal sleep time, and now you may have a hard time getting your infant to go to sleep, so sleep may also be short. That, despite your best efforts, will make it very difficult to have a routine to your day. Getting the right timing for the onset of sleep can relieve stress during sleep time and can also facilitate longer duration of sleep, both during daytime and nighttime.

Soothing strategies

A large proportion of the babies are unsettled. Some find it difficult to sleep without parental intervention from some low to medium to high rates. They recognize that in the sense of sleep, the ability to be autonomous of parents may not develop until six months plus, and may not emerge spontaneously even at that age, but need to be strengthened and developed.

Try not to worry about what you might consider as' bad habits' - in the early days there is no such thing. Do not take much notice of good-meaning suggestions that you' make a hook for your own back' or that your kid is' playing you.' From a nutrition and growth standpoint, there's so much going on that your baby needs a strong level of support from you, then you have to give it and do so guilt-free, because it can eventually diminish, or you'll be able to reduce that as they get older and they're more open to learning.

If this sounds familiar, focus on improving coping mechanisms rather than wondering if your baby is unsettled. If your baby struggles — would like to be up and on you, which is very typical — develop a lot of ways to help them relax, other than just eating. Teach them how to respond to a variety of soothing steps.Assist the needs of your infant with plenty of support-try different positions. Babies are major gesture lovers–they wantbouncing in your arms or (safely) bouncers and chairs. Attempt not to get stuck with just one way to calm your baby–the more you can calm your baby, the simpler it becomes to phase out agitation and unusual resting positions as your baby grows older.Do not be afraid to use a pacifierin the early days, especially if sucking helps to calm them down.

- Introduce only on establishment of food.
- Never dip in sweet syrup or teething gel or medication.
- Ensure pacifiersare always clean.
- Evade the use of loops or cords to protect pacifiers.
- Do not be scared! This need not be a long-term commitment.
- Baby slings and wraps
- Infant bouncers
- Pram / buggy
- Rocking in a rocking chair
- Traveling by car
- Vibrating chairs
- Bouncing on an exercise ball.

Where will baby sleep?

Ultimately most babies are going to sleep in a conventional cot, but generally not until they're six months plus, because at the beginning a cot may be too big a space.

A Moses basket or a crib that can be put next to your bed (this is called a cosleeper or sidecar) are probably the best choices for nighttime and even some day-sleep. Usually this sleeping room is temporary because the baby gets big fast and then maybe transitions to a traditional cot. There are plenty of choices on the market and there are even a few that make the transition from a newborn sleeping space to a kids bed. Don't be overwhelmed; your choice will be based on your budget and room, and your priorities and parental style, of course.

Your baby will probably share a room with you for at least the first six months.

Instead, they can move out into their own bedroom depending on the rooms available and your own feelings about where you want your child to sleep.

- Your kid will take advantage of a small space to start feeling healthy.
- Young children sleep better and longer with their mums.
- You'll always have to invest in a new mattress for every new child. And keep this in mind if a family or friends send you or borrowed a Moses basket, crib, or cot.

The mattress has to be solid, compliant with health regulations, and you should always put the baby close to the end of the crib with its feet.

- You'll always want your baby next to you during the day and in the evening. Theymay at first have a propensity to sleep wherever and whenever with noise and light that doesn't really disturb them.

- Your buggy's pram part will act as a creche very well. The baby can lie flat and be relaxed, and if you don't schedule a stroll, you can always roll them in the house to help them drift off to sleep.

- Your kid will have a late bedtime to begin with, so you'll probably keep them in the pram living area, your arms, or the Moses basket with you. You will all go to bed when it's bedtime and the baby will be in the crib or Moses basket for the night (in theory at least).

- While you may not plan to share your bed with your baby, there is scheduled and unplanned bed-sharing and nothing wrong with it. You shouldn't feel guilty about this sleeping approach; yes, it can help a lot of mums get more sleep. Although it is not supported by the current health agenda, it would appear that at some stage as many as 70 percent of parents share the bed. So if you're sharing rooms, whether expected or not, make sure you practice safe sleep and provide a risk-free environment. Even if you're sharing the bed, that doesn't mean that you can never change the conditions. Consider returning your infant to the cot once they're 12–16 weeks old in addition to reducing their expectations of sharing your room.

Quality sleep in the family bed

There's no one way for your family unit to handle healthy sleep. There are many different styles of discipline and essentially it's a personal choice. Infant sleep can be hotly debated and controversial indeed. Decisions about where your baby will and should sleep are deeply personal and your opinions may change depending on your infant.

For many couples, co-sleeping –also referred to as family bed or bed-sharing–can be a wonderful, integrated solution and can work exceptionally well. Some parents, however, feel that although they have no problem sharing beds or cosleeping with their family, no one gets much sleep. That still doesn't mean you have to give up sharing the room, it can only mean you have to review the situation and make some adjustments to ensure things work a bit easier.

Second, as with any solution to sleep, you have to practice healthy sleep. Adult beds have not been built with safe sleep in mind and parents have to make sure the space is safe. Infants will sleep on their backs, under breathable, comfortable bedding on a solid, clean sheet. Families will avoid loose bedding, stuffed toys to pillows and make sure the baby doesn't get too hot or cold. Stop using a mask to get your baby to sleep. It is imperative that there are no holes or spaces that threaten crushing or suffocating your baby. The surroundings should be free from smoke. Links to smoking is one of the most prominent risk factors in SIDS.

Never take the chance that you fall asleep on a couch or armchair with your baby. When you feel very exhausted and think you should sleep with your kid while nursing or cuddling them on a couch or armchair, move to a bed–keeping in mind the safety guidelines–or, when possible, ask your partner, friend, or family member to take care of them while you get some rest.

Ideally, both parties should be involved and consulted before beginning to bed-share.

Everyone who shares the bed should agree with this family-oriented judgment, and also understand that everyone who occupies the bed is responsible for the child's health and well-being. Clearly it is not advised to use caffeine, medications, or medicine and those unable to wake quickly should not co-sleep with the baby.

SIDS rules recommend that parents should postpone co-sleeping for the first three months, or if the baby was born before 37 weeks, or weighed below 2.5 kg/5.5 lb.

Nevertheless, as this is the most natural environment, many parents will co-sleep much earlier, particularly when breastfeeding is completed. Personally, with my full-time (11 days over!) 8.6 lb bundle of joy, I committed to this practice and it meant we all had a lot of sleep.

If there's a question, consult with your GP or health-care consultant. In the first instance, using a' sidecar' or' co-sleeper' attached to the main bed can very often be a very good alternative. If you are feeding, it is preferred that the baby sleeps with the mother on a different sheet, rather than in the crib, so the'sidecar' is the option here.Note, there is no proper sleeping path. It must be the right thing for you, and it must be safe and free of threats. Whatever you choose, it can be modified and perfected to make it sleep-enhancing for everyone involved as well. For those first few months, parents should do what feels right and then you can look at things again when your baby is older and more open to being apart from you–if that's what you want.

Establishing a bedtime routine

The baby will start smiling back at you from six to eight weeks of age.It means they are adjusting to social cues and so it's a perfect time to start doing a pre-sleep routine, one that makes them realize that sleep time is what comes next. It also lets the kid cool down before going to sleep and takes them from alert to sleepy. Once you have developed it,you can also use this routine before nap time.

Reference routine at bedtime

1. Twilight
2. Switch Night Nappy / Dress
3. Sing songs in series
4. Use some slogan, for example ' sleep time, boy '
5. Provide feed to bedtime
6. Put the baby in its sleeping room.

The percentage of wakefulness approach

This method helps to develop the ability to sleep. To encourage the ability to rely less on parents during the'going to sleep' process, put your baby in the cot, more awake than asleep, specifically at bedtime. Sleep problems may begin to appear when your infant is six months of age or older if they have not developed the ability to sleep without parental intervention. At this early stage, you have the perfect opportunity to avoid ever having a dependency-based sleep problem.

Some babies come to get through the day with a high need for support from you.

They do arrive, though, built to do some of the hard work in sleep time, but only if you give them space and motivation. Youneed to be careful, encouraging them to become part, if not completely, aware of you as they grow older at sleep time.

Bedtime, although late, is the best time to first exercise and develop this skill set. Try to avoid getting your baby to sleep at bedtime, and encourage them to do some of the work of falling asleep. This may be the next positive step in ensuring long-term sleep difficulties are avoided. Initially, your baby may beasleep 100 percent before you put them in their bedtime sleeping space.

Once you have started to get a sense of regularity to the day, and understand the language of your baby's sleep, and have developed a pattern of bedtime, the next step is to try and make them sleep less than fully at bedtime. I am referring to this as the percentage of wakefulness, because most of us can see what 100% asleep looks like and in effect can see what 95% asleep and 5% awake would look like as well!

Get your kid to the point of sleepiness and start putting them in the crib until they sleep fully. Gently comfort them with physical support such as touching, stroking, and soothing them, and emotionally encourage them with shushing or soft humming, whether they fuss and squirm and whine a little bit. If your baby's getting increasingly agitated, pick her up and get settled back to sleep and try in another day or two. When you continue to work through this process, they will slowly-and particularly at bedtime-become more aware of being put down especially consciously entering a resting environment with less interference from you. You are, therefore, laying a road to a sleeping capacity that will work in your favor as time goes on.The premise is you're moving through the process, but you're not going to continue if your kid isn't patient and is screaming desperately for comfort and support.

Dummy tip

If you use a dummy, you can try to weaken the dummy's association with sleep, thus reducing the need to re-plug countless times by practicing removing it before your baby sleeps completely in their sleeping space. If your baby roots for the dummy, when they are rooting, push the chin up; if they get upset, return the dummy and repeat as many times as necessary until your child goes to sleep without it.

Again, you may need to judge the effectiveness of this approach, as it can sometimes be a frustrating exercise for all!

Some gentle natural solutions

Teach your kid the distinction between day and night over the first four to six weeks by using daylight and waking time exposure to light and using dark lighting for nighttime. This will help regulate the body clock and continue laying the groundwork for safer and faster sleep. Parents may start seeing a daytime structure appearing beyond 10–12 weeks of age, and may look forward to longer stretches overnight. When baby gets older the need to differentiate between day and night becomes less important and thereafter I recommend a dark space for all sleeping as the body makes the difference naturally.

Get plenty of outdoor and fresh airplay. Studies support young infants who sleep better and longer than those who do not sleep outside, especially in the afternoon.

There is a suggestion babies are more active in the light, and light influences the biological clock's early development. This regulates many body functions, like sleep hormone melatonin secretion, which plays a key role in well-balanced sleep patterns.

Enable as muchdaytime sleep as indicated by the temperature. Do your best to ensure your baby is well-rested all day long. Do not panic if your kid is only going to sleep on the go or in arms-this is a good strategy in the short term-the more rested they are, the more they can sleep at night. When baby is older and more open to learning, they can work on phasing out the motion sleep.

Keep your child near you. Room sharing is recommended for the first six months, but, as well as the advantages of decreased SIDS risk, research also shows that staying next to mum will control the sleep patterns of the infant. Night feeds can also be achieved with low noise.

Use white sound. The vibration that imitates the womb/heartbeat or the sound of a clock, extractor fan, or hairdryer will soothe baby immediately. Don't use real devices (for safety reasons); you can download apps or buy CDs. Do not use white noise that has turned too loud for an extended period of time, and move the device away from the ear of your baby. Don't underestimate the quick capacity to stimulate and then control the heartbeat, raise the alpha waves in the brain, and actually help the baby fall asleep faster and deeper. If your baby goes to sleep listening to white noise, this should remain on for the entire period of sleep. Do not think about wanting it for the long term; by slowly turning it down, you can wean the baby off.

If you're not with your baby, use a baby monitor for peace of mind. Decide on the one that best suits your family and then make sure that it'sat least one meter away from the baby.

Learn to treat children. Atnight, infants that aremassaged fall asleep more comfortably and into a deeper sleep. Massage can also enhance digestion, growth, and development along with the sleep benefits as well as provide a perfect bonding opportunity.

Although your baby doesn't seem to like it, make sure that you keep encouraging tummy time from six weeks on throughout the day! Commit each waking hour to 5 to 10 minutes. Be imaginative and use the floor or crib (supervised) to get your kid to move. I really like to see this ability develop after four months and it will help the infant relax; they can get comfortable and sleep in a natural position.

Reflux and intolerances

Reflux and milk intolerances may be one of the biggest challenges for a young infant's mother. A reflux baby can be much more than a problem with laundry. For many parents, it can be a living nightmare, with situations varying from moderate to severe. In the first few months, as many as oneout often infants will be affected, although many will outgrow itwithin 6 to 12 months. Seeingthe pain and discomfort a baby may feel with this condition can be difficult, leaving parents frustrated and drained as they try to seek answers from a variety of sources. If you are worried that this disorder willaffect your infant, please seek advice from a health care professional. A combination of medication and interventions from a wide range of sources, such as formula changes, adjustment of the diet of the breastfeeding mother, cranial osteopathy and sacral therapy, and feeding and sleeping positions, can manage a lot of cases.

Reflux and intolerances can have a significant impact on your baby's sleep, to make things even more stressful. Once these problems are controlled, there's usually no reason why your baby can't go on to be a great sleeper; it can just take extra time as you discover the extent of your baby's problems and because of the reflux you may be left with unhelpful sleeping associations. Many reflux babies also have food sensitivities and food intolerances, which can further wreak havoc on healthy sleep; common symptoms, including pain and discomfort, can be really regular nighttime waking, restless sleep and/or long wakeful stretches overnight. You will have to work closely with your pediatrician,

GP and visitor to health. It may be impossible to expect the infant to sleep through the night or for any length of time until the problems are handled and properly under control. In the meantime, you can try to create a framework for getting better sleep soon and surviving the reflux roller coaster.

1. Use the guidelines pertaining to age eating and sleeping. Don't forget the waking suggestion no later than 7.30 a.m.,so you regulate the body clock and align your daytime feeding schedule. A baby with reflux may benefit from feeding little and often, but make sure that you anchor the day within 30 minutes of waking with your first feed to avoid sleeping and feeding clashes all day long. Feeding less, and often, can make the situation worse at times. Although it seems to help your baby cope, it can also mean that they never take a full feed and therefore you never manage to get into a daytime schedule that is appropriate for aging. It would be preferable to get the symptoms under control and then pace and balance your feeds and sleeps properly throughout the day. If you provide medication, do so immediately upon waking so as not to delay any further feed.

2. You can then help plan when sleep should occur with a regular timetable. Babies with reflux may be more difficult to read than other young babies. Early sleeping symptoms may not be that clear and you might do better to focus on the clock time. Beware of the early signs of getting tired– brief eye rubbing, yawning, and zoning out. First thing, the wakeful period can be quite short, with some babies

under the age of six months requiring a nap within 45 minutes of waking up–this is obviously made harder if you have to keep the baby upright for 20–30 minutes after feeding. It can mean you have to firefight all day with an overtired and refluxing baby, allowing overtiredness to occur first thing in the morning. I would suggest that in most babies up to eight months you try to prepare for a nap within a maximum of an hour and forty minutes of wake-up. Keepinga sleep log, which can help identify the right times for sleep, may be helpful. When you think it's time to sleep, take your baby to a quiet/dark environment to help them relax and their signs of sleep may become more visible.

3. Talk with your doctor or health visitor about sleeping positions. Babies who are distressed may not rest well on their backs, despite supporting the'back to sleep' prevention campaign for SIDS. Try to sleep the kid on the left side once they're old enough to do that. Look into a wedge or other service items that can be of assistance.

4. Practice lots of tummy time, despite any outcry. Do this often; it will help develop the ability of your infant to roll back and forth onto their tummy, which in turn, helps them to sleep comfortably. This promotes the ability to become comfortable without input from parents.

5. Raising your cot. You may also need to create a little nest at your baby's feet to stop them from slipping down; and, of course, keep safe sleep at all times.

6. If your baby is very irritable and things are very rough, don't think about where the daytime sleep happens, just try to make sure it works – buggies, bikes, slings, and swings can all help your baby calm better even if they're not 100% relaxed.
7. Make sure you're grooming the kid to sleep comfortably. Consider using relaxed waist tops and sleepwear.

Reflux Signs and Symptoms:

- Frequent voming, both by mouth and sometimes by nose. Be conscious that not all children are constantly vomiting; some have a passive reflux, which means the acid comes up, causing pain, but no vomiting.
- Some reflux babies may be slow to gain weight but not all.
- Willingness to feed, or at least remain on the job. Often eager and then arching away from the breast or the bottle, causing disturbance to the feeds, or needing little and often milk.
- Constant hiccups, chokes, or gags.
- Sour air.
- Chronic irritability, prolonged crying in the day for long periods.
- Inconvenience while sitting on the bottom.
- Sleep disorders, constantly awakening, sometimes clearly in pain.
- Chronic coughing/cough.

To help you get to the bottom of these things, see your doctor or health care provider. You'll be able to build better sleep if controlled.

82

CHAPTER 7: NAP TRAINING

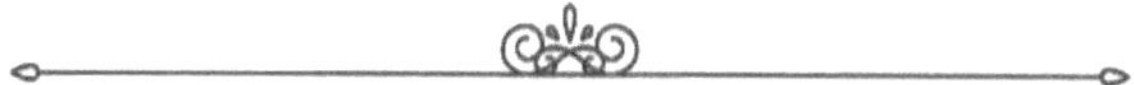

If parents just want to encourage their baby to sleep through the night, but also want to continue to nap them on the go, or even though they are already sleeping during the day, they will almost always find that it is only a matter of time before their child starts to struggle to fall back asleep during regular sleep cycles.

Because there are so many variables involved in naps, and because it can take some serious finessing to get them right, we think naps are an art. Nonetheless, the possible obstacles are worth jumping over, as the willingness of your child to nap well will have a profound impact on her ability to sleep well at night.

Why isn't my child napping well?

Poorly spaced naps are the most common cause of brief or irregular naps, mainly because young children have such a tiny window where they are exhausted enough to sleep long enough, but not so overtired that they wake up from the nap too early. We'll cover comprehensive schedule details according to age in this segment, but feel free to skip to your child's section.

A word of warning about naps: they're much harder to fix than nighttime sleep, so please don't be frustrated if you see fast and (relatively) simple nighttime progress but notice that you're dealing with the naps a little longer. There are three main reasons for tricky naps:

1. Children's bodies aren't as exhausted as they are after a full day at night, so it's more challenging to fall asleep and stayasleep.
2. Children are mindful of the sunshine outdoors, and don't want to slow down their bodies or interrupt what they're doing to sleep.
3. During the day, children love to spend time with loved ones and familiar carersand they don'twant to be apart from you for a while.

Even though nap challenges take a bit longer to fix, if you execute the schedule closely, your child will learn how to snap back quickly. Consistency in how you react to your child when he/she develops is, as always, key to your success.

When you help your child adjust to a new nap schedule, you'll find that he/she sometimes seems a little distracted when he/she develops her new skills, maybe not even getting a full hour for every nap. While we warned against allowing your child to get overtired, we need to help her nap well at the right time and allow her to stay awake long enough between sleeping periods during the day, he/she can both fall asleep and stay asleep for a total of one hour. When helping your child adjust to their new nap schedule, stretch it as closely as you can to the next sleep period without allowing her to get exhausted. Babies under the age of 6 months will usually have a harder time waiting all the way until the next nap time than babies over the age of 6 months do.

How many Naps does my child Need?

Until you commit your child to nap training, first determine how many naps they need every day. The numberof naps a child needs usually corresponds to their age, but here the term "every child is different" applies.

Four to seven months

For general, a four-to seven-month-old child should be napping three times a day. If they are awake from7:00 a.m. approximately until 7:00 p.m. Scheduled naps will take place at 8:30 a.m., 11:30 a.m. and 3 p.m. For feedings, every day after waking in the morning and after each nap, the last feed takes place half an hour prior to bedtime. Most children in this age range already eat at least once overnight, so feeding them should not be needed more often than at these times.

Sample schedule for a three-nap baby:

- 6:30-7:00 a.m.: wake, milk feeding
- 8:30: nap
- Wake, milk feeding
- 11:30: nap
- Wake, milk feeding

- 3:00 p.m.: nap
- Wake, milk feeding
- 6:30: final milk feeding, bedtime preparations
- 7:00: bedtime
- 1:00 a.m.: night feeding

Remember, that no times are mentioned when the baby will wake from every nap. Using the time a baby has been awake (i.e., "wake times") to determine when they should next sleep can cause chaos in the life of both the baby and the parent. If a baby takes a nap of any duration they should be put to sleep as close to their next scheduled naptime as possible.

Seven to Fourteen Months

Kids in this age range usually only need two naps a day, about 9:00 a.m. and 1:30 p.m., if the timetable is 7:00 to 7:00 It is imperative that the second nap starts at 1:30 p.m. so the distance between nap two and bedtime is as short as possible. Also, if still breastfeeding or bottlefeeding, try feeding after wake-up in the morning, after each of the two naps, and half an hour before bedtime. If your child still does not regularly eat solids, consider adding milk at around noon to another meal. If your child is eating solids, plan to feed them breakfast about an hour after waking up in the morning, lunch at noon, dinner about two hours after waking from their second nap (which should be about two hours before bedtime). Most babies should not need a nocturnal feed unless the pediatrician of the child has stated that they still do.

Sample schedule for a two-nap baby:

- 6:30-7:00 a.m.: wake, milk feeding
- 8:00: breakfast solids
- 9:00: nap
- Wake, milk feeding
- 12:00 p.m.: milk feeding or lunch solids (it is especially easy for baby to become drowsy during this milk feeding due to its proximity to naptime, so work hard to keep your child fully awake)
- 1:30: nap
- Wake, milk feeding
- 5:00: dinner solids
- 6:30: final milk feeding, bedtime preparations
- 7:00: bedtime

Fourteen-month-old toddlers usually only need one nap every day from about fourteen to eighteen months, beginning sometime around11:30 a.m. At 1:00 p.m., at lasting between one and a half hours and three hours, depending on the boy. A child who takes one nap each day usually gets all or most of hiscalories from solid foods and liquids (milk, etc.) through a sippy cup. Nutrition times can be changed according to need. Unless your pediatrician advises otherwise, the provision of a milk feeding half an hour before bed is probably no longer required. Sleeptraining books make it easy to determine, but how many naps are best for your child can be difficult to decide.

For the babies of four to six months, begin with the assumption that three naps are required. If they are particularly willing and fall asleep twice during the day, consider moving down to two naps even after ten to fourteen days of nap training. While your child can benefit from three naps, if they don't allow themselves to fall asleep that many times a day, learning to integrate all their day-to-day sleep into just two will be their responsibility. Conversely, maybe you've got a four-and-a-half-month-old who regularly naps two hours each morning, making it hard to cram in three naps every day. Rest assured that even if they're just taking two naps, your baby can get all of their required sleep each day.

If your child is between seven and fourteen months of age, usuallythey require two naps each day. This holds true in almost every event, at least through their first birthday. Nearly all children go through a period of about ten to eleven months, often lasting up to a month, during which theyreject one of their naps every day. Eventually, parents start to think that fighting a nap (usually two naps) is a sign that their child needs only one nap each day. This relapse appears to go through within one to two weeks, so parents shouldn't change their everyday habits. Once your child reaches the age at which moving them to one nap is acceptable, you should seeif their behavior meets one of the following criteria:

1. Your child is over age 14 months and has regularly battled one of their two naps for two weeks straight or longer each day.

2. The child naps comfortably twice a day, but fails to fall asleep every night before 9:00 or 10:00, or starts to wake up in the middle of the night.

A notice on scheduling: About 7:00 am for most babies and families until 7:00 p.m. It seems that plan works best. If your family canmanage a 7-to-7 schedule, I encourage you to make an effort to follow the nap times listed below. Some families are unable to adopt a 7-to-7 schedule for a variety of reasons, or may simply feel their child will flourish at different times with naps and bedtime. Do what you find works best for your family and baby, applying these nap training techniques as regularly as possible, so don't be discouraged either way.

Nap training can be very difficult. This requires a significant amount of parental engagement and resilience and it will be extremely tempting to deviate from the methods described below. Generally speaking, parents can focus on one to two weeks of naptraining. Parents must start the morning after the first night of sleep training in order for the nap training to be successful. Many babies immediately take to nap training; some need a few weeks. It takes at least one week for it to really last, in most situations. Many babies may seem to be sleeping well in the first few days, only to struggle with naps on day three or four. This is presumably because they made up for lost sleep during the first days of training, and the real training has only begun now.

When baby is down, they'll have an hour to try to fall asleep. There are only three possibilities within that hour.

1. Baby falls asleep for less than forty-five minutes. If this happens, instead of running right in when you hear them rouse, give them ten to fifteen minutes to try and go back to sleep (the only reason they woke up after all was because they had finished one sleep cycle and had trouble entering the next). When baby falls back to sleep, get them up the next time they wake up, and make sure they don't sleep for more than 120 minutes throughout the whole nap. Note, don't count crib time, count real asleep time. When baby doesn't fall asleep again, get them up after ten to fifteen minutes and feed them instantly, making sure they don't fall asleep or become drowsy. They should be kept awake, no matter how short the nap was, until their next scheduled naptime (review the previous section to proceed with the sample schedule).

2. Baby falls asleep and is sleeping past the 45-minute mark. Thismeans that your baby has completed one full sleep cycle and has moved successfully to the next one! Anytime baby wakes up, get them up, feed them, and go on with the day, between minute 46 and minute 120. Do not encourage your baby to sleep for more than two hours during a single nap, and always make sure there is a difference of at least ninety-to-105 minutes from the end of your nap to the beginning of the next. For rare cases, babies sleep so long during their first nap that they cannot fit in a third nap, which finishes at 4:00 p.m. If this occurs, consider doing just two naps that day, with the second beginning at

1:30 or 2:00, holding the bedtime at the same time or changing it to30 minutes earlier.

3. Baby refuses the full hour sleep. In this case, you should get baby up and feed them immediately (because it's been about three hours since their last feeding), while making sure they don't fall 100 percent asleep while eating. Thirty minutes later, settle them down for another one-hour nap. If the baby went down at 8:30 a.m. for instance,and they did not fall asleep for the full hour, they should get up at 9:30, feed, and keep awake until 10:00, and then put back down for another one-hour nap attempt, during which they will either take a short nap of less than 45 minutes, a long nap of more than 45 minutes, or no nap at all. Follow the above instructions according to which situation arises.

You'll want to set aside the value of a plan as you go through the first few days of training, and instead concentrate on the following guidelines:

- Start your infants' day at 6:30 a.m. to 7:00 a.m.
- Aim to start nap one as near to 8:30 a.m. as much as possible.
- Do not require the baby to have a nap after 4:00 p.m.
- Do not put them down again until the next scheduled naptime, or as close as possible, if the baby gets some amount of sleep for the nap.

- Similar checks are appropriate during night training, but remember that for many children, contact during nap hinders their attempts to fall asleep, so avoid checks during naps if possible.

A notice on feeding: if you're going to feed your baby when they wake up from every nap attempt, they're going to eat every two-and-a-half to three-and-a-half hours a day. So before a nap I would be highly wary about feeding them again. In most situations, when a parent thinks a baby is hungry close to naptime, inreality the baby is simply tired, which is why they fall asleep so quickly when milk is provided. You want to break the link between eating and going to sleep. That said, you are the only one who has the special ability to decide if your child needs a feed or not. If you need to feed your baby sometime other than right after a nap, make sure they stay fully awake throughout the entire feeding cycle.

It's very necessary for your child to be awake when they're with you, and just fall asleep when they're in their own crib. However, sometimes it'll feel impossible to keep your baby awake in the first few days of training and particularly with younger babies. They might even fall asleep while playing under a gymnasium! If your baby sleeps peacefully outside their crib, let them stay asleep and don't move them. Perhaps turn off the lights inside the room and put a white noise machine near where they sleep. Control them and let them sleep as long as they wish when following the above guidelines. When they wake up again, go on with the rest of the day, ensuring their last nap doesn't end until 4:00 p.m.

Two naps

Nap training all kids hasmany similarities, so be sure to read the outline for three-nap babies before you start with your two-nap kid's process. Luckily, the fewer naps an infant takes, the simpler naptraining seems to be. Older babies are usually better at handling less daytime sleep (which is normal in the first days and weeks of nap training) than younger children.

Get your kid out of their crib from 6:30 a.m. to 7:00 a.m. and give them an immediate meal. When they eat solids, give them breakfast about an hour after waking. At around 9:00 (or any time before 10:00), go into their room and use the five-minute calming method to put them down. The baby will also get an hour to try to fall asleep, but we won't concentrate on their nap duration.

1. If, at any point, your baby sleeps and sleeps for any amount of time, get them up as soon as they wake up and give them a milk feeding. Keep them awake until their next scheduled naptime (1:30 p.m. or later) or as close to as possible. Instead, if you think a nap is too short, you should wait around 10 to 20 minutes to give the baby a chance to fall back to sleep before they get up. When they fall asleep again, get them up the next time they wake up and do not allow them to sleep for more than 120 minutes total.

2. If your baby doesn't fall asleep for the hour, get them up and feed them with milk (keeping them fully awake), and

put them down for another one-hour attempt thirty minutes later.

If they take naps at 9:00 a.m. or 10:00 a.m., and again around 1:30 p.m. or 2:30 p.m., you may get into a tricky situation if your baby doesn't sleep on their first attempt, and then sleeps on their second attempt. When they take a nap around midday and it takes seventy-five minutes or more, then decide if it makes sense to offer them another nap. When you think they will fall asleep again and wake up no later than 4:00 p.m., give baby a one-hour nap at least 3:00 p.m. However, if your baby sleeps at around noon for the first time and lasts until about 2:00, they probably won't be able or willing to fall asleep again before they have to be up by 4:00. You can do an early bedtime as early as 6:00 p.m. in this case, and be consistent the next morning by beginning baby's day no earlier than 6:30 a.m.

As for three-nap babies, the same rules apply: stay home for the first two to four days, no napping past 4:00, no single nap longer than two hours, and check-ins are fine as long as they do not appear to make the baby more agitated and upset.

One nap

Nap teaching a child who needs only one sleep a day is a double-edged sword. On the one hand, kids tend to handle missing a nap fairly well, but on the other hand, they can choose to skip a nap for weeks, battling naps every day and not allowing themselves to nap for several days in a row. Fortunately, as with most other babies, most infants take to nap training within the first ten days. Also, reading through the nap training method for babies on three and two naps will be useful, since both of these examples provide relevant details for babies with single naps.

Milk is probably no longer the primary form of nutrition for your toddler, so making sure your baby gets enough calories is a little simpler. Provide them with breakfast, and maybe a snack a few hours later, after getting your child up for the day between 6:30 and 7:00 a.m.

Beginning from 11:00 a.m. to 11:30 a.m., put your child down for an attempt using the same five-minute relaxation strategy mentioned above, again allowing them an hour (or up to ninety minutes if you believe your child will benefit from more time trying to sleep) to try to fall asleep on their own. Check-ins are almost always harmful at this age, so it might be best if you allow your child to be alone during their attempt. If your kid sleeps for any length of time, get them up as soon as they wake up, and keep them up. If required to accommodate a quick or early nap, please feel free to move bedtime earlier by up to an hour.

If your kid isn't sleeping, then give them up to two more attempts. Here is a sample training schedule:

- 11:00 a.m.-12:00 p.m.: nap attempt one
- 12:30-1:30: nap attempt two
- 2:00-3:00: nap attempt three
- Early bedtime if no successful naps

When they fail to sleep throughout the day, be especially careful they do not fall asleep before bedtime. Babies who only nap once a day should have up to three hours of sleep, but naptime will end no later than 3:30.

How to transition to fewer naps

Once you've finished sleep training, a time will come when you need to shift to fewernaps. Your child may get tired throughout the whole process once you make a move. That's natural, so if you're certain that your child is ready, according to the guidelines below, don't let their tiredness prevent you from reducing the number of naps you need.

Three to two

The change between three and two can be tricky to navigate. But, your child will be ready to go down to two naps when they are:

1. Not falling asleep for all three naps (because nap three isn't exhausted enough);
2. For all three naps, falling asleep but unable to fall asleep at bedtime or waking at night or early in the morning, unable to return to sleep; or
3. Can fall asleep three times a day, but the last nap is so late it will go past 4:00 p.m.

Just put your child down at 9:00 a.m. when you decide it's time for a change to two naps and 1:30 pm, and if you need to, go to bed earlier. Generally, the process takes just seven to ten days, so stay consistent and don't go back and forth between three and two naps.

Two to one

Know that it will be about thirty days before they combine all their day-long sleep into one nap when it comes to changing the toddler to just one nap each day. Do not throw in a second nap over this long period of a month just because the daily nap of your child was only forty-five minutes. Keep them awake until bedtime, maybe putting them down 30 minutes earlier than normal, but don't go back and forth between one nap and two.

In this era, it's fairly straightforward to change nap schedules. You can always go cold turkey and keep your child up until about 11:00 a.m., put them down for a nap, and then keep them awake until bedtime. I recommend changing kids slowly, shifting their first nap of the day to around fifteen minutes later every two or three days, while continuing to put them down about 4:00 for about thirty minutes. Every day (on the presumption that they're not going to sleep, just "rest" in their bedroom with the lights off and white noise on). Stop putting your child down in the afternoon once the first nap starts at 11:00 but keep moving the 11:00 nap slowly later until it ends at what you deem the appropriate time for your child (about 12:00 to 1:00 p.m. for most children).

Step by step sleep for naps

Implement those rules once you have hit your allocated nap time. You will use these same methods whether your child has never napped well or if you are trying to lengthen a short-nap habit.

You will give your child a minimum of one hour practice time in the crib or bed for each nap, whether he/she is sleeping or not. It counts per minute so try not to give up after 50 or even 55 minutes. We have met many kids who at the very last minute ended up falling asleep! If you leave your child for the full hour in her room, he/she will have a good chance he/she needs to learn how to put herself to sleep.

You will continue expanding your child's time in the crib or bed with kids napping once a day until he starts sleeping close to an hour. For starters, if he's learned how to sleep 50 minutes, consider encouraging him to stay for 90 minutes in his crib or bed to help him start to lengthen the nap. If he doesn't seem rested after learning how to sleep for 90 minutes, prolong the length of the nap by increments of 30 minutes.

Step 1: Prepare Your Sleep Station

Just like you did at night, get your station ready for sleep. Remember this station is critical to correctly monitoring your plan. If you forget what you are supposed to do and inadvertently deliver inconsistent or mixed messages to your child, he will sleep less and cry more. Writing down all the information throughout the learning process becauseyour infant will also help you see improvement from sleep to nap. Noting his gradual improvement will also allow you to stay motivated to achieve your goals.

Mind Your Verbal Baby about Sleep Changes

When you continue your nap time schedule, go over with your child her new sleep rules again and read your special sleep book (just like you did at night). Remind her that the night before he/she did a great job and now he/she will practice falling asleep for the nap. Let her know that he/she will feel refreshed after nap time is over, and that you can play together. Reminding your child of the program will make her feel more empowered and thus more able to participate.

Step 2: Do a Mini Version of Your Bedtime Routine

Do a mini routine in the same room where your infant sleeps, just like you do at night, before the start of the day. What you're doing for naps doesn't have to be the same as what you're doing at night, but every nap should have the same nap routine. Check your Sleep Planner to make sure you've made all the environmental changes required for your child to snuggle comfortably.Remember to ensure that your child does not fall asleep under the same old conditions that he used to (such as rocking or feeding or staying in the room). If your kid is used to falling asleep on the breast or bottle, take him off the minute you start to see the symptoms of "drunken sailor"; heavy eyelids, slow-down breathing, and rapid loss of consciousness. Grant him a little twitch when this happens: "Honey-honey-honey! We're not yet able to fall asleep. "Crack the window and get some fresh air in.

Allowing him to sleep for even a moment will take away the edge of his tiredness, keeping him from being able to nap at all.Put your child in your dressing room or bedjust like at night, wake up your child and say, "It's time for nap, sweetheart! See you early." Then, leave the room.

Step 3: Do Your Check-Ins

Record the time you put your child in bed at hersleeping station. Now you're going to start helping her lovingly while she tries to sleep just like you do at night.

For Crib Sleepers

Do your check-ins at the same time that you used for the night, remember not to contact your child; keep the check-ins short, 30 seconds max; and try not to go any sooner than the check-in period so your child will have enough time to sleep. If the check-ins make your child cry harder, it's okay to extend check-in intervals for naps, waiting as long as you feel comfortable. Remember to record it all in your sleeping station.

Key Points to Reduce Protest Crying

1. Wait for the same check-in time you've scheduled.
2. Do not contact your kid if he/she feels taunted whenever he/she's crying seriously, let the noise reduce before you check on her.
3. Use a cool, affectionate tone of voice to inspire her.
4. Live max. 30 seconds

For Bed Sleepers Not Using a Gate

If your kid gets out of bed, instead of checking in, say, "Oops, you got out of bed — let Mom (or Dad) walk you back." Put him down, and leave the house again. Continue to walk your child back to bed every time he or she leaves the room— which may last the entire hour as your child begins to work on naps— without talking (which is too stimulating for your child during the day and will make it more difficult for him to fall asleep). Remember to remain calm, as any reaction from you— even slight frustration — will only reinforce the protest and continue.

Key points to raising opposition as your child is going back to bed

1. Do not allow yourself to be drawn into conversation with your child, which will give her incentive to remain awake and cause her to protest for longer.
2. Do not give in to water requests, a kiss, and the like. During your wind-down cycle, you will have already provided these.
3. Do not express your anger or frustration with your child, which will strengthen herbehavior. If you need to stop, let the other parent take over.
4. Every time you return your child to bed, leave the room quickly.

Step 4: Praise Your Child's Hard Work!

Whether he/she is asleep or not, I would like to congratulate your kid for her outstanding efforts to learn how to nap. Older kids who grasp your words will be very proud of their accomplishments!

Gauging Your Child's Nap Progress

Your child will learn how to go back to sleep for naps in just a few days, without screaming or complaining.

Though, once your infant continues to learn how to sleep, he/she will likely fall into one of the three groups below:

1. **THE PROTESTOR;** throughout the hour your child can weep or protest. Don't be afraid! During the first few attempts to make improvements in naps, this can happen. As frustrating as this can be for both you and your kid, note that he/she is studying learning how to sleep (or, if older, learning new rules), even though he/she is still not completely pleasing. He/she is going to get there soon!

Solution: If he/she doesn't sleep at all, at the end of the hour, wake her up and give her lots of praise anyway, reminding her thatshe was trying hard. Kiss her as much as you want, hold her, cuddle her. Pause for an hour (for infants under six months of age) or until the next nap time (for children above six months of age) and start again.

2. **THE PENDULUM;** In this case, the infant may scream a little, then sleep a little, then weep a little bit more — in other words, he/she may sleep off and on over the course of the hour. This may be normal in her first couple of napping attempts, when children may just sleep enough to take the edge off and then wake up, still fully relaxed.

Solution: No matter how much he/she has slept, if he/she's waking up at the end of the hour, get her dressed. If after a few days of working on naps you want to try stretching the nap a little longer, you can try to keep your baby in her crib or bedroom for an additional half-hour, and when he/she wakes, poke your head in the door and say, "Always nap time sweetie. Go to Bed!" When you have removed your child from her bed, keeper up until the next scheduled nap time.

3. **THE PROCRASTINATOR:**your child may cry for a significant portion of the hour (including 59 minutes!) in this scenario and then sleep. Hooray, he/she's done it!

Solution: Let him/her go forward and sleep as long as he/she likes, up to 2 hours from the moment he/she slept.

Wake him/her up after 2 hours; if he/she is going to have another nap, keeper up forthe appropriate time period before the next nap.Always, make sure he/she gets up early enough to be able to get safely down before bedtime. Children who nap once a day can sleep for 3 hours.

Working on Naps Can Be Exhausting!

When you feel overwhelmed by all the efforts being made to improve the ability of your child to sleep, you are not alone! The bulk of the communities with which we work share the same feelings. When you find that the challenges of your infant day and night are just too much for you to bear right now, and you ask if you can put the naps back later to fine-tune, the answer is yes. Though your kid will not have consistent practice in practicing his new sleeping habits while you split focusing on nighttime and nap time sleep, the brain will manage night sleep and day sleep differently, so you can continue to enjoy satisfaction with the adjustments you're making at night to keep helping him/her sleep through the day.

If you have a baby sleeping with a motion— car or stroller — these options are superior to sleeping over breastfeeding or rocking, but if the two are your only choices, go ahead and use it. If you're not going to work on naps for now, try helping your kid get as much nap sleep as possible and focus on night sleep.Make sure he/she's not exhausted by bedtime (which will cause higher cortisol levels and more crying). If your child is unable to nap well no matter what you do to help him/her, it is best to move forward with naps and learning.

The Emergency Nap

If you've tried to help your child nap well several times a day, or if your child has only gotten fragmented nap sleep on a given day, put him/her in the car or stroller and let him/her take a nap (preferably at least 1 hour) with movement. That way, he/she won't get distracted by bedtime, which will make it harder for him/her to fall and stay asleep. If you have the choice, the use of old habits (such as breastfeeding, pacing, or lying with your child) to help your child sleep is preferred.

CHAPTER 8: NIGHTTIME SLEEP TRAINING

The age of children being taught to sleep in a bed varies widely, from as young as seventeen months (usually about when some kiddos climb out of the crib) to as young as three-and-a-half years. Although older children may be educated in sleep, these approaches are intended for those who are three-and-a-half and younger. Unfortunately, the most difficult period for sleep training is between seventeen months and two-and-a-half years, because younger children cannot recognize many of the strategies used to induce older babies to choose to stay in their rooms and go to sleep. If you need to train a child in that range and find it hard to keep them in a crib, I would strongly suggest studying methods to safely prevent your child from getting out of their crib before trying to train in a bed (make sure your doctor is fine with any strategies you might want to try). Many parents succeed in going from a crib to a Pack' n' Play, because the mesh sides make it more difficult for babies to climb up and out. Many first confirm with their pediatricians that it's okay to put their children in sleeping bags to encumber their legs so they can't climb out of their crib. If your kid still climbs out of his or her crib, read on.

First, you'll need to plan the sleep environment for your kids. It should be 100% childproof, with all the furniture— dressers, bookcases, changing tables — bolted or secured to the wall (well, earthquake straps). I've heard of kids scaling furniture and toppling them down, hurting them or even worse. Any other risks, including anything that a child may choke on or tie around their necks, should be removed. Get down on your hands and knees and make sure there's absolutely nothing your child can get on with that could harm them. Also, be prepared for the possibility of your child attempting to turn off the lights by removing the bulbs from the overhead lights and even taking lamps with you once you say good night. Finally, dress your child so they can't take off their clothes and/or diaper. Try cutting off a footed sleeper's feet and placing it on backward so your child can't take it off. As with younger children, make sure that you use loud white noise to ensure as much silence as possible in the nursery and watch your child with a video monitor at all times. Finally, in the first few weeks of training, many children tend to sleep on the floor instead of in their crib, so leave some bedding (a sleeping bag and pillow is normally enough) by the door if that's where your child wants to sleep.

You will need to be prepared at some point to keep your child in their space by more dramatic means, including a gate at the door, a protection doorknob cover for the kids, or a doorknob with a lock facing the hallway instead of the bed. Most parents are balking at the thought of "locking" a child in their room but don't worry about confining them to a crib. In terms of keeping a kid in a completely safe position (their bedroom), it makes more sense to think of it just as if you kept them in their crib. The real safety problem around this age is when not only is a child unable to fall asleep unassisted, but they can also leave their bedroom at will. Toddlers are exposed to all kinds of dangers when they have the freedom to come and go as they please, and are more comfortably confined to a bedroom than getting the middle of the night free range of the house.

Of all the options available to keep your child safe in their bedroom, I highly recommend that you choose the cover for the doorknob. A gate may seem more humane, but typically it only compels a child to stand at the door for long periods of time while they scream into the house to get your attention. A lock is effective but unnecessary; it works equally well with a doorknob cover. Especially with older children, they seem to get upset by a cover less than a locked door. I recommend switching to a doorknob for your child's room if your doors have levers as handles, because the commercially available handle covers for knobs are much more convenient than the ones available for levers. Consider investing in a toddler clock that lights up a certain color every morning when it's time to start.

Finally, choose one of the following ways to show your child how many chances they will have to choose to stay in bed until the morning. The former will work best for kids who like to sleep with their door open, and the latter is better for kids who like to sleep with it closed.

For children who like to sleep with the door open, open the door of your child's bedroom until it hits the threshold at an angle of forty-five degrees and put a piece of masking tape directly below the door above the floor. Open it about one-fourth of the way up to the threshold and put another piece of tape, another one-fourth with a piece of tape, another one-fourth with a piece of tape, and place one last piece of tape at the threshold itself (where the door is closed). There should be a minimum of five pieces of tape, marking the door open at an angle of ninety degrees, then at markings 1/4, 1/2, ¾, and fully closed.

Children who prefer to sleep with closed doors should have four sticky notes placed high up on their door side. The final preparation is to create a large, colorful sticker chart on a poster board, with columns representing days, and rows representing every conceivable activity you do with your child before going to sleep, starting with dinner (i.e. baths, pyjamas, books, kisses, etc.). Usually add all the things that your child asks for as reasons for trying to leave their bedroom, like a drink of water or using the potty. This isn't a typical sticker chart in that finishing the chart doesn't profit. Rather it acts as a family visual checklist.

Don't speak with your child about those plans. You'll later explain what it all means, but playoff the importance of these changes if your child sees them before beginning sleep training.

Present your child with the chart at dinner on the first night of training, exclaiming excitedly that you will be using it before bed from now on to make sure you do all the things you need to do before going to sleep. Don't say anything about sleep training or "staying in bed"— just act like that is a nice, new thing you're trying to do, and make sure you're using stickers that are going to be especially appealing to your child.

It's time to start after dinner. Start at the top of the map, and work down your way. Do not focus on anyone while you go through every operation. For example, when you ask your child if he wants a sip of water, ask, "Would you like a drink of water?"If they ignore you, or don't respond, ask them again, this time adding," Would you like a drink of water? If you don't take your chance now, that's it; you won't get another chance until the morning."Irrespective of their reaction or failure to respond, add a sticker to the map and don't go anywhere. Also, don't be too particular about the stickers— if your child wants one for everybody on the map on his shirt, that's okay. If your child later asks for a drink of water, let them know they've had their chance; then, leave them in their bedroom with a sippy cup of water so they can get access to it overnight.

Once you've done all of your bedtime activities, explain clearly to your child that from now on you're going to sleep in your bed until morning and they're going to have to stay in their room, in their bed, until morning. Make sure your child understands this while not dwelling on it any longer than necessary. Show them the clock of the toddler and explain that when it illuminates it means it's time to start the day. Explain the tape marks on the floor at this stage, or the sticky notes on the door. Tell your child that if they get out of bed once, the door will be closed to the first mark (or the first sticky note will be removed), and the door will be closed or you will delete a note for each time they leave their room until the door is closed all the way or the sticky notes are all gone.

Explain then that when the door is closed, "it will remain closed until the morning," when the clock goes off. Do not show the toddler doorknob cover to your child or explain how it works, or that they cannot open it. If you are using the sticky method, make sure you leave the door almost closed but not closed all the way after removing each sticky note, since you want to allow your child to practice their ability to actually open the door so that once the door is closed, they understand that they need to remain in their bedroom until morning. No matter the reaction of your child, work hard to stay calm and rational. Give your child a hug, tell them that you love them, leave the room and follow the directions once they go. Leaving their space and losing their "chances," calmly walk them back to bed, telling them that you love them and that you will see them in the morning. It is important that you remain happy and rational through this training process, and never give in to complaining, cajoling, pleading, or fighting. Just move the list down, and proceed to bedtime.

A small number of kids need only one or twodoor closures or sticky note removals before they decide to stay in their rooms... often while they throw a fit. Do not continue to take away their chances by closing the door in stages or by taking away sticky notes as long as your child remains in their room. I've seen kids fall asleep over the door threshold with their heads, and their parents and I counted that as a win! It doesn't matter where they go to sleep as long as your child remains in their bed and falls asleep unassisted. If your child exhausts all their chances at bedtime, the door must be shut and left closed until the morning. Do not communicate or talk through the door with your kids, and give them no more chances. Watch them through the monitor closely, and let them be, as long as they remain safe. Keep the door shut until the clock goes off. For hours, some kids have been known to cry or protest, but the vast majority of the time, if you apply this method exactly as outlined, kids will only take thirty to sixty minutes to sleep. If your child uses a few opportunities, then he or he/she falls asleep, only to wake up and leave their room in the middle of the night, resume wherever you are, walk them back to their room and take away one of the opportunities. Nodrama or talking, just lay them in bed again and move on.

As with all aspects of sleep training, the most important job is being consistent at every level. The fantastic thing about teaching infants to sleep is that they usually get it, and quickly! Nighttime training sometimes takes only one or two nights, and then you're done, assuming you're doing nap training concurrently and being consistent in ensuring that your child sleep entirely unassisted.

Nap Training

The name of the game is endurance (and, as expected, consistency) when it comes to naptraining. Over the first three days, approximately eighty percent of babies can adjust to nap preparation, with the remaining twenty percent going on a full nap strike for up to seventeen days. Stay strong... Stay strong! If you're consistent, toddlers can start napping; stay the course, and allow the cycle time.

Because kids are taking only one nap each day at this point, you're going to perform up to three one-hour nap attempts every day, making sure your kid doesn't fall asleep in the car or anywhere else other than the bed while they're working on learning to sleep at home consistently. As with crib training, do not start sleep training until your child can stay at home for the first forty-eight to seventy-two hours of sleep training 100 percent (with no outings for any reason).

I'd suggest making your first attempt about 11:00 a.m., depending on the time your child usually naps. And midday. Put your child down for a nap using the same chart and door/tape or sticky note form, and allow them up to an hour to fall asleep. If they struggle, get them up for a 30-minute break, then put them down for another hour again. Make one final attempt if they are still unsuccessful, then keep them up until bedtime. If at any point they fall asleep, then get them up as soon as they wake up alone. Even if the nap is short that day, don't try any more naps. You may find that when given two ninety-minute attempts instead of three one-hour attempts your child does better. This is also an effective form of nap therapy, as it allows kids a bit more time to try to fall asleep alone.

It is very, very important that during sleep training you never allow your child to fall asleep in any other place than their bed. Don't give in and encourage them to take a nap, because they need a "break" and couldn't fall asleep. One of the Baby Sleep Trainer Method's secrets lets the body re-regulate its own daytime sleep. The only way to interfere with that cycle is to require or enable your child to sleep in the car or stroller, or anywhere else other than their own room.

If your child spends the day in daycare, you're in luck! Toddlers in daycare sleep very well, almost without fail, even if on the weekends they snap badly at home. Generally speaking, it is the "mass mentality" of all their sleeping peers that encourages them to go to sleep alone. I'd encourage you to do weekend nap training to encourage your child to sleep well when they're with you too.If your child is not napping anymore, continue with nighttime training and miss the nap training altogether. Note that a toddler's sleep training is almost always going to come down to some sort of standoff. Be strong for your child, and provide the support required in your home to help them become the successful independent sleepers they need to be. If you've suffered months or years of poor sleep, realize that sleep training will actually take less effort than anything you already do, and will culminate in giving your child the precious gift of having all the sleep their bodies really need to develop, learn and thrive!

CHAPTER 9: NIGHTTIME FEARS

Most kids occasionally feel scared at night and fears can lead to problems with sleep: scared kids don't like being alone.I will outline a number of useful considerations in assessing the severity of your child's nighttime anxieties, and describe methods you can use to address them. Although professional help may be necessary for a very anxious child, by using such techniques as emotional support, desensitization, rewards, schedule adjustments, negotiation, unlearning of automatic behavior, and limit setting, you should be able to manage most of the anxiety-related sleep problems yourself.

The Anxious Child

He/she will face many new challenges as your child grows. During the day, he/she needs to learn to handle being apart from you—alone in a house, with a sitter, or in daycare, nursery school, or kindergarten — and (at some point) every night when he/she goes to bed. He/she has to learn how to controlhis/herbehavior, bowels, and bladder; hold in check the feelings of anger, jealousy, and aggression; and master the give-and-take of interacting with family and friends. He/she is going to learn, wonder and maybe worry about death, God, heaven, and hell. They may love sexual pleasure but may be anxious about masturbation. He/she will doubt his/her ability to perform on a par with her colleagues, and wonder if he/she can live up to his/her expectations.

Every stage of the development of your child brings with it particular vulnerabilities to some anxieties.

Forstarters, her fears about separation can escalate for a while when he/she starts nursery schooling.

During the daytime he/she may be reluctant to leave your side and may not want you to abandon him/her at bedtime. He/she may feel guilty if you get sick, imagining that his/her angry words or thoughts caused your illness and made you less accessible to him/her than usual.

Training in toilets presents other concerns. Your child might be worried about herability to control herself.

Yet he/she could be drawn to dust. Yet he/she wants to please you at the same time, and he/she may be afraid to incur your disappointment. Such issues are heightened at night for many toddlers; how can they prevent soiling or wetting while they are asleep?

A scary movie can be particularly frightening for a 5-or-6-year-old. He may be very disturbed by abduction scenes, or those where a child displays violence against an adult. To a boy, the films can be very real. Both children have violent dreams, and most feel a little bad about them, but it can become a source of great fear to see these feelings play out on the television.

Although the ages of six to twelve are known to be a period of relative social stability, children between infancy and teenagers face pressure in a number of areas: education, athletics, music class, worship services, home, and even from their own minds. Children are struggling to make connections and find new role models apart from their parents; children are called upon to become more confident and more open to home issues; and they are starting to carve out their own identities. At these ages, previously unrecognized learning and psychological issues can become obvious.

Most kids sleep alone in this age range. A child too scared to do so may be embarrassed to lether friendsfind out. He/she may not be able to take part alongside his/her friends in events that require staying away from home overnight, and may feel him/her self-confidence shattered and his/her self-image deteriorate.

Adolescents, too, when they experience the sudden physical and emotional changes of puberty, and struggle with major concerns. They are beginning to worry about the future-college, jobs, money. Sexual feelings for teens are very strong. Moral issues are becoming more common, and as teenagers deal with new and important choices, they face constant dilemmas. In areas such as academic performance, sexual habits, and drug and alcohol use, they must weigh personal desires against peer pressures and family standards. We can experiment with new systems of value, and abandon old ones. They may feel their parents are no longer accepting or loving them and they may completely reject the assistance of their parents.

Many teens with worries severe enough to influence their nighttime sleep choose to struggle alone rather than calling for help from their parents. These young people need help, but they may be more able to get that help by therapy than the coping approaches discussed in this book.

Bedtime Fears

Anxiety is a frequent and important cause of problems in bedtime and nighttime wakings. It is relatively easy to keep preoccupations under control during the day. Most kids have too many things to do, and too many distractions to sit and brood. But even a child who feels pretty comfortable during the day can feel insecure at night. He/she may begin to worry, waiting for sleep to come. There is little to distract his/her mind, as he/she lies in bed in a cool, quiet room, so his/her ideas and imagination will run free. When he/she wakes up in a dark, quiet house with everyone else sleeping during the night, his/her anxiety may get even worse. It's a small wonder that even a child who doesn't have any difficulty going to school can resist going to bed at night in his/her room.

Because the ability to control one's thoughts and feelings diminishes as one is exhausted, children sometimes come back at night and start feeling and behaving more immature. In that situation, a five-year-old may need the same amount of reassurance during the day as a three-year-old does. Scolding him/her or telling him/herhe/she's being a baby won't help. Perhaps trying to figure out why he/she feels insecure. He/she may need you to be more engaged in his/her care at such times than you might be during the day.

While some anxieties are normal, or at least reflect inner struggles that are part of normal development, others are caused by external events. Every significant social disturbance that the infant has little control over— illness, parental conflict, breakup, or divorce; obesity, or other substance abuse; death — can give rise to much distress, shame, anxiety, and terror at any age. When a child has to give up what little influence he/she has over her life at night, along with the ability to remain aware of what's happening outside her house, hallucinations triggered by these strong feelings are especially likely to emerge, and they can be quite frightening. Hardships and worries at bedtime are to be expected.

Evaluating Your Child's Fear

Not all night-time "scared" reports mean the same thing. Many kids talk about fears when they're not very worried at all; others are really scared. Many kids are only terrified of insects; some tend to be frightened of everything. Some are just terrified at bedtime; others are similarly frightened all day long. That is why not all concerns about being scared at night should be treated in the same way. You might find it helpful to consider the following questions when deciding what kind of support your child needs.

Is Your Child Really Frightened?

1. He/she looks scared when he/she says he/she's scared and acts scared? If kids wake up their parents at night, they usually explain themselves by saying "I'm afraid" or "I've had a bad dream." But it's easy for kids to say they're scared whether or not they are. Such words can be pronounced by rote and without much real meaning. If, in a matter-of-fact manner, your child reports his/her "fear," and if he/she's calm and doesn't seem scared, then he/she's not really scared, in all likelihood. In this case, gestures are more accurate than words. The complaint may be just one of many that your child has tried; he/she may have dropped requests for extra drinks or tuck-ins and started complaining in his/her room about "monsters" because that complaint is the one that has the best results. As a parent you don't want to respond to this "pseudo-anxiety"; it's only encouraged by your response. On the other hand, if the anxiety is sincere, you do want to respond.

2. Is he/she experiencing such bad dreams? Kids now and then have dreams, but if your kid says he/she has a bad dream at night, note that hallucinations typically only occur rarely and are not usually the cause of constant nighttime disruptions. Most kids who talk regularly about bad dreams are unable to explain much about the hallucinations, mostly because there wasn't one. After a really scary dream a kid will look and act in terror, and he/she will have to tell a real dream tale (unlike a vague reference to "monsters" or "bugs" or "robbers"). The child's fear,

as always, is measured more by paying attention to how he looks and behaves than by the particular words heuses.If your child wakes up very frightened by a frightening dream, he/she shouldn't have to stay alone; but you probably want to avoid sitting with him/her every night. You will help him/her self-orient and understand he/she's not in any real danger. It can also help byactually discussing the dream.You can do that quickly at the moment, but the next day is best for deeper talks (discussions in the middle of the night will rapidly become a bad habit).

3. Shouldhe/she measure limits? It is important to distinguish a child who is anxious at night from one who is only testing limits— the appropriate responses are quite different— but it's not always easy to make this distinction. An anxious child and one testing limits are both likely to resist going to sleep, make additional requests at bedtime, call out repeatedly, and keep coming out of their rooms. Both may speak of anxiety (remember, any reason seeming to work will be used by a child checking limits). For extreme cases, it is easier to tell the difference; the nervous kid seems to be very afraid, while the limit tester may even chuckle.

Therefore, the more aggressive you get with the frightened child, the more scared he/she becomes; a limit-testing child may get upset (not afraid), or his/her actions may just change.

Limit-testing issues and anxiety often arise simultaneously, because improper setting of boundaries can lead a child to become afraid. Children need proper, predictable, consistent boundaries and their absence can lead to anxiety growing. When parents happily give in to additional requests on some nights and thenthey respond with frustration and threats on other nights, then the child will not know what to expect. He/she may want to askanother question but he/she will be understandably nervous about your response. Here's a situation where setting reasonable nighttime limits for an upset infant will help matters, whereas if the fear has a different cause, strict limits are likely to make it worse. If you're not sure that the key problem is poor setting of limits, err on the side of assuming the anxiety is caused by another cause. The limits can always be set later.

4. He/she just isn't sleepy? If the issue with your kid is fear, then heshould sleep fairly quickly in the evenings while you are together (if it is obvious to him/her that you will be together all night). If it takes him/her too long to fall asleep there with you, then he/she might go to bed too early. As explained in Chapter 9, in the hour or two before the time we usually fall asleep we all go through a period of extreme wakefulness.Many children forced to go to bed too early behave like children with limit-setting problems; they keep on calling their parents with various excuses coming out of the bedroom. Some very well-behaved children (perhaps too well-behaved for their own good) stay put, but they may lie in bed without the option of reading or watching tv, fantasize, and eventually end up scaring themselves. Under such situations, even though they are not intrinsically nervous people, these kids do get a bit

anxious. The anxiety vanishes when the bedtime hour is adjusted.

How Severe Is Your Child's Anxiety?

1. How strong are hernighttime fears? You need to determine just how pronounced her anxieties are at night to help a child with anxiety-related sleeping problems. Observe the behavior of your child, again— don'tjust listen to his/her words. When a child is really terrified at night it is usually obvious. When bedtime arrives, he/she gets scared, even terrified. He/she'll be clinging to you, crying and begging not to be alone. He/she can accept any punishment as long as he/she isn't going to have to stay alone. He/she cries from under the covers when he/she wakes up at night terrified of losing his/her house, or he/she runs to your room. If instead he/she finishes gathering his/her blanket and teddy bear before walking quietly to your room, and then waits politely by your bed waiting for you to wake up, he/she may be a little anxious, but it is doubtful that he fears will be severe. A frightened child may move into your room at night, but if the fears are very intense he/she won't go back to sleep on your floor without first waking. The worries of a child can't be very serious if she can comfortably go to sleep in the evenings when you leave him/her with a sitter. Likewise, the more nervous a child becomes, the less likely it will be to want (or be able) to sleep in a

friend's house. A very frightened child may face humiliation even during sleep in his/her own house, leaving his/her friends in his/her room to join his/her parents in theirs.

2. 2.Was she feeling anxious all day or just at night? Anxiety which is present throughout the day is more worrisome than anxiety which only appears at night. If you find that your child has no difficulties during the day at home or in daytime programs, and that he/she is social, enjoys being with others, and is not easily panicked you should be reassured. If this is the case it is likely that nighttime fears will be isolated and easy to deal with. But if, throughout the day, he/she appears anxious about many things and in different settings and activities, then it is less likely that the nighttime anxiety can be resolved simply and by itself; instead, more general psychological assistance may be indicated.

3. Is he/she having trouble breaking up in the daytime? Separation anxiety is normal in kids but can appear at virtually any age. It can start at approximately eight or nine months of age. A periodof heightened anxiety sometimes lasts several months and then slowly eases. A child with separation difficulties is unlikely to be left with a sitter easily, and he/she may still be up and awake when you get home; he/she appears panicky and cries every day when he/she is brought to daycare or pre-school, and the panic doesn't quickly disappear when you leave; he/she resists going to school; and he/she refuses to sleep with friends, or calls to come home. When you're out of the house with

him/her, he/she may refuse to leave your side, and maybe reluctant to join in activities or play with others, even if you're close by. At home, whenever you leave the room, he/she may get frustrated even for just a few minutes. If he/she has these problems with separation, it could be unfair and unrealistic to ask her to sleep in a bed by him/herself. On the other hand, even if he/she's really "clingy" at home, you should be encouraged if you notice he/she's doing well with sitters or daycare (at least once you've left), doing well with others, and not afraid to try new things. If he/she handles separation well during the day, and especially if he/she goes to sleep without a problem when left with a sitter, you can rest assured that he/she can handle separation at night.

4. Is itlongstanding anxiety or is it a recent evolution? A terrifying video, something heard at school, or a bad dream may cause anxiety over the short term. Transient anxieties such as these affect all children and do not indicate a need for professional advice. For parents, encouraging and caring both at night and during the day, these anxieties usually overcome themselves within a couple of days or weeks. A child with occasional fears will find the extra compassion offered by parents very helpful during those fearful periods.Just knowing that such help will be available when it is needed can reduce the severity of these fears and shorten their duration.

Long-standing concerns are a cause for more worry, lasting many months or longer. Such fears will reach into a child's day and influence her behavior choice. If severe, the probability that the child will have difficulty coping with normal daytime activities increases. With support alone, such fears aren't likely to disappear. Bear in mind that a frightening film seen once does not usually cause huge, permanent scares, but it can unmask already-present anxieties. Consequently, even if long-standing anxieties are traceable to a traumatic case, the real cause may be quite different from the original catalyst.

What Is Your Child Afraid Of?

1. Is there an external cause for his/her anxiety which can be identified? While single events such as a scary film mightreveal underlying anxieties, they may also cause short-term problems and long-term worries— if exposure becomes repeated or continuing. There may be a specific reason for the apprehension of your child; a television show last night, a family illness, or the absence of a parent because of a business trip. At school, he/she may fear a bully, an unsympathetic teacher, or an upcoming test. Or the root of the anxiety might be trouble at home (maybe parental fighting, alcohol, perhaps depression). You may be able to provide sufficient assistance with understanding and support depending on the nature of this cause, or you may need to seek professional counseling.

2. Does it seem as if he/she's scared of many things, or is he/she just scared of a few specific things? As a rule, some

kids aren't scared but have significant fears about particular things, such as insects, spiders, snakes, or fire. If the source of terror turns out to be rain, as with Tyler, the child may only have sleep problems on stormy nights. You need to make yourself particularly available to him/her on those nights; if you refuse to comfort him/her at those times, he/she may get scared every night, worrying that there will be a frightening storm and he/she'll have to get through it alone. For example, in order to address the concerns of mosquitoes, spiders, snakes or flames, you should educate your child through talking tohim/her about the steps you have taken to avoid them (or, of snakes, that there is none where you live), or by slowly desensitizing him/her by schooling (using books) and observation (at zoos and museums). Yet, most importantly, if there is any question, you must convince her of your ability to protect him/her.Unless, however, your child is frightened of many things, day and night, he/she might have a more common form of anxiety. Unless those fears are mild and manifest only rarely, it is impossible to overcome them by trying to deal with the coping strategies listed below. Professional therapy would possibly also be needed here.

3. Does he/she fear the "monsters" and "robbers?" If your child develops distress symptoms he/she doesn't grasp, he/she'll typically use her imagination to come up with an explanation. He/she has to consider something that he/she can assume to be a source of her worries, something external and dangerous that he/she has no power over: ghosts

and robbers. These anxieties are normal especially in young children.

They often concern control issues related to toilet training, hostility towards a new sibling, or the need to keep aggressive impulses in check at daycare or preschool.

Remember that while the predators or thieves aren't real, the terror of your child is true. This originates from real feelings, desires, and fears. He/she doesn't understand that these emotions are what make her nervous. Your child doesn't need safety from predators to overcome these fears: he/she needs a better understanding of her own emotions. If she spills, has a temper tantrum, or gets angry at her brother or sister, she needs to know that nothing bad will happen. She can be better encouraged at such moments by understanding that you are in care of yourself and - to the degree that she wants it - of her, and that you can and will defend her. If you can persuade her of these issues he/she'll be able to relax more. Because these monsters represent the feelings of your child, not things in the room, your tranquil, firm, and loving assurances will do more to banish the goblins than searches under the bed. Spending half an hour of flashlights behind the furniture every night does little to reassure your child, and it may even reinforce her fears: why would you look so hard if monsters couldn't be there? The monsters are in your child's mind and you should concentrate your efforts there. He/she certainly needs reassurance; if he/she wants more than that depends on how frightened he/she is.

4. Is he/she concerned about the dark? No kids like to live in complete darkness and there's no need that they should. It is helpful if the bedroom is dimly lit by nightlight or streetlights from outside, so that when your child wakes up at night, especially after a dream, he/she can see where he/she is, reorient herself inside the room, restore a sense of reality, and put the dream in its proper perspective.Usually a nightlight (two to seven watts) suffices when a child is afraid of the dark only. But an anxious child might ask for extra lights: first a table lamp, then an overhead light. The space always ends up illuminated very brightly: a minimum of between 60 and 200 watts are popular. Many parents turn off the lights after their child sleeps, but when he/she wakes up in the dark, he/she gets scared and turns the lights back on or a parent has to come in to do it for her. Others leave the lights on all night. But even 60 watts are very bright at night (as we all know, our eyes adapt to the dark at night and become more sensitive to the light; if we explain it to them, most school-age kids can understand this too). Waking in that much light is a heavy stimulation of anticipation which is not conducive to a quick return to sleep.In reality, a child rarely prefers darkness to the shadows created by a nightlight. That's good if it's her choice and if he/she sleeps well without any sun, in truth. But for some children, the fear of "darkness" is the same as the fear of monsters— that is, the terror does not exist in the shadows, but the child seeks to rationalize it by blaming it on something else, causing an insecurity that

he/she does not understand. If the clouds go out he/she will have something else to fear.

5. Is he/she afraid to have her door shut? Just as most kids want some light in the house, so, at least at night, most want to keep their doors ajar. It applies especially to scared children, though those whose fears take the form of thieves may actually feel better when the door is closed. The open door generally allows a child to have a sense of connection (to what's outside), awareness (to where her parents are), and reality (to where he/she is). Hearing her parents move about or watching local tv is comforting, as it reminds her they are there. He/she could use her imagination to determine, the same creativity that conjures up demons, once the door is closed and he/she can't hear what is actually happening outside. Don't fear her night will be disturbed by the normal sounds of family activity. If he/she only gets scared when her door is closed at night, the remedy is easy.

6. Does the fear have a self-reinforcing pattern? Most often, when an isolated event like a scary film causes a child to get scared at night, the fear will last no more than a few weeks. However, sometimes the nightly memory of being scared, and perhaps of the inappropriate responses of her parents to the fear, leads to increased anxiety that spirals out of control until the child reaches a state of near panic.Each night the infant remembers the terror of the previous night, not the initial cause.Suppose a child wakes out of a genuinely frightening dream one night, wakes up

her mother, and discovers that they are waking up with rage, warnings, and punishments. He/she is now as frightened of their reaction as of the vision. He/she's afraid to go to bed the next night, because he/she knows that if he/she has another scary dream he/she won't be able to get help, and he/she also knows he/she might get so scared that he/she's going to have to wake her parents up, which will only make them angrier. The fear of their getting upset with heradds to her distress. If the next night goes poorly, her anxieties can intensify until the nighttime transforms into a fight for her parents, and a time of fear. Whatstarted as a single bad vision becameweeks or months of tremendous chaos. The parents and even the kid may have forgotten the initial vision at that stage and have no idea what he/she is actually scared of. No one gets enough food, the parents get frustrated, and the child suffers badly.

When I see a family at this juncture I always consider the possibility that the underlying problem may be less serious than it appears, even though everything seems out of control and the child is terribly scared. The spiraling process can be reversed with proper interventions, and the escalated fears gradually brought back under control. The child's experience of falling asleep quickly and without fear is of utmost importance, so the only bedtime memory the next night is a good one, and the spiral may become one of increasing trust. Then, and only then, can it be decided whether there is a significant psychological problem which predisposes.

How to Cope with Nighttime Fears

If your child is not really scared: Like most parents, you might be able to tell if your child is really scared. When you realize he/she doesn't really look scared or behave that way, you need to be strong. Stay with the routine of bedtime, and say good night. Do not go there again and again. See Chapter 5 for more guidance on setting clear boundaries and helping your kid comply.When you make this decision, be as confident as you can. If an infant is actually scared at night, it won't help to be strict in this way. It could escalate matters.

For Very Mild Fears: If your child starts having trouble going to sleep because he/she's worried or somewhat frightened at bed-time, talk with her over the day. Be empathetic and compassion-ate at night and be helpful. As long as her worries are relatively mild, you should probably not make any significant changes to her bed and night routines. You might sit in her room with her a little longer than usual, but keep her on her normal schedule as much as possible (except, perhaps, to set her bedtime for a while later than usual, as discussed below). Just reassure her firmly and calmly that he/she's safe and you'll take care of her; then put her to bed with her usual story of silent talk. In the long run, your child will be more reassured if you show her you can take care of her than if you give in to her anxieties.

For More Substantial Fears: If your child is anxious at night and has more than a few mild worries, the number one goal is to do whatever you need to do to remove the anxiety. Other problems could also be addressed. Therefore, all the recommendations below follow the same basic formula: Begin by doing whatever it takes to help your child feel comfortable and able to sleep well during the night— but aim not to do more than required. When things calm down, gradually decrease the extra support and raise the trust of your youngster at a pace he/she can handle.

For a child with mild anxiety, even very small steps can be of benefit. Keep in mind that the anxiety could be the product of a cycle you need to undo. The better it is every night the easier it will be the next night. Try to keep to more or less the same schedule and routines as before, particularly if the fears have recently developed. Be sure to find daytime and evening time for your child. Pleasant and unrushed should be the bedtime routine; understanding and reassurance are important. At least initially, try to determine how much support your child needs to feel safe and secure, and offer it freely. He/she needs to know he/she can get help without getting you angry or upset. That knowledge alone makes the evening less appalling.

Every child is different but some of the techniques described below will be helpful for most children at least. The strategies first listed may be appropriate to help a child with moderate fears; those later listed may be necessary for children with more severe anxieties.

CHAPTER 10: PICK SLEEP SOLUTIONS

Read through all the ideas and note those you think could help your reference. Prepared with your solutions, you can then begin to follow your personal plan. Solutions for

Newborn Babies— Birth to Four Months

Congratulations on your newborn baby. That is a moment of glory in your life. Whether it's your first baby or your fifth, you'll find this a time of healing, change, sometimes disappointment and frustration but, most happily, falling in love. Newborn babies have no problems with sleep but their parents do. Newborns sleep when tired, and wake when able. When their schedule clashes with yours, they do not have a problem; they don't even know it.

During the first few months, the activities you do will set a trend for the next year, or two or more. During the next few months you should take steps that will help your baby sleep better. You can do this in a gentle, loving manner that does not require any weeping, tension or rigid rules. Babies less than four months of age have very different needs to apply certain general ideas than older babies over the next few months will set the stage for better sleep over the years to follow.

You should start using those suggestions for older babies when your baby hits age four months. Nevertheless, if you read, understand, and apply the following tips for newborns when your baby is still a newborn, this book may not be needed when your baby is four months old. Isn't that a great thought?

Read, Learn, and Beware of Bad Advice

Clearly everyone has an opinion on how to raise an infant. Remembering how many people felt compelled to share their wisdom when my first child was born, I was shocked.

The threat to a new parent is that these tidbits of misplaced advice (regardless of how well-intentioned) can really have a negative impact on our parenting skills and, by implication, the growth of our children, if we do not know the facts. The more experience you have, the less likely it will make you question your parenting skills.

My goal, and that of the other respected and knowledgeable parent educators who share the bookshelves with me, is to present the facts as we know them, so that from the constructive power of information and not the reactive weakness of ignorance, you can choose the method. In other words, if you're aware, then you're shielding yourself and your family from the onslaught of "should" and "would" that don't suit you or your family, and may even have no evidence or facts to support them. That is the game plan I was inspired to create by an interesting conversation with my single, male, childless friend. I realized that my friend's opinion would have left me puzzled, worried and self-doubted if I had not been educated and assured on this particular issue. He has managed to make me speechless, at the very least. So, it's intelligence that is your best defense. It is, as they say, real power. It's the sun that illuminates ignorance in the dark halls (or cribs, in this case). The more you know, the happier you'll be forming your own child-rearing philosophies. If you have the facts straight, and if you have a parenting plan, you will be able to respond confidently to those who are well-meaning but give counter-or incorrect advice.

So, the first step is getting smart! Know what you do, and know why you do it. Then, you can smile when those amateur experts share their advice, and say "Wow, really? "And then go about your business in your own way, with quiet confidence. The marketplace contains a number of outstanding books on children. I suggest reading a baby book or two, and building your information shop. As you read, keep in mind that no author will 100 percent parallel your beliefs, so you have to learn to take the ideas that work best for your family from each one.

Sleeping Through the Night

You have either read or heard that at about two to four months of age babies start "sleeping through the night." What you have to remember is that a five-hour stretch (the one I described be-fore) is a full night for a new baby. Most (but nowhere near all) babies will sleep uninterrupted from midnight until 5 a.m. at this age. (Not that they always do.) That means a scream far from what you might have imagined sleeping through the night! Here we pause for those of you who have a baby who sleeps through the night but didn't realize it, the shock sets in. If your baby is already sleeping through the night, then next time the old child-birth education group meets, enjoy the heady pleasure of brag-ging rights. What's more, while the scientific definition is five hours, most of us wouldn't take that anywhere near the sleep of a full night. Sometimes, some of those sleep-through- the-night people will suddenly start to wake up more often, and it's often a full year or even two before your little one falls into a normal, all-night sleep routine every night.

Where baby wants to sleep

Where does your baby feel most secure and comfortable? In the body. Where is your most happy baby? In the body. Where would your new baby tell you he/she'd like to sleep if given the choice? Yeah, in your arms! Nothing— absolutely nothing — is as en-dearing and beautiful as a newborn baby sleeping in your arms or on your breast.

Maybe it's because mothers are conditioned biologically to crave their babies in their arms.

But — threat WARNING! Look out! A baby who sleeps in your arms will always want to sleep in your arms— you guessed that.

Smart kid! A baby who cries for the protection of the arms of her mother or father, and the parent who responds, operates within the natural instinct system that has helped ensure the survival of babies from the beginning of time. That very real and all-consuming bond will work perfectly in a perfect world— where mothers do nothing but care about their babies that whole first or secondyear of life. A world where someone else manages the house, prepares the meals, provides the means to pay the bills— while mommy and baby spend their days loving each other and doing those good, bonding things that nature intends. Alas, if ever it did, such a world no longer exists. Contemporary life does not provide this luxury, with its demands. Mum has a lot to do and we have to strike a balance between passion and practicality.

A Forward-Thinking Suggestion

So, I hope you'll learn from my error as hard as it may be. Put him down in his bed when your baby is asleep. Nonetheless, don't fully deprive yourself of the precious joy of baby sleep. Do enjoy this treat from time to time. But unless you think you can spend hours each day with a two-year-old on your lap, you'd better let him get used to sleeping in his crib. The idea of sometimes putting your baby down alone for sleep is extremely important to those of you who choose to co-sleep with your baby. Babies require far more sleep than adults do. I've worked with a lot of mothers whose babies are so used to Mom's presence in bed that Mom has to put herself tobed at 7:00 and stay there because her baby's radar is built-in andwon't let her leave him alone. Mommy will take daytime naps too, whether he/she likes it or not! The intention is to enjoy your baby's co-sleeping moments but also show him that he can sleep alone.

Falling Asleep at the Breast or Bottle

To fall asleep while sucking on the breast, on a bottle, or with a pacifier is very common for a newborn. Yes, some newborn babies do this so naturally, and so often, that mothers are worried they cannot eat enough. When a baby still sleeps like this, he begins to equate sucking with falling asleep; he cannot fall asleep any other way over time. A large percentage of parents dealing with older babies who are unable to fall or stay asleep are battling against this normal and efficient suck-to-sleep relationship. So if you want your baby to fall asleep without your support, it's important that you sometimes let your newborn baby suck until he/she's sleepy, but not fully asleep. Disable the breast, bottle, or pacifier as often as you can, and let her end up falling asleep without putting anything in her mouth. Your baby can resist, root, and fuss when you do this to retrieve the nipple. Giving her back the breast, bottle, or pacifier is perfectly fine, and starting over a few minutes later. Repeat. Replicate. Replicate. He/she will eventually learn how to fall asleep without sucking if you do that often enough.

The next step in this strategy is to try to put your baby in his bed when he is tired, rather than sleeping. A sleepy infant, too young to have ingrained habits, will often embrace being put in his crib or cradle while still awake, and then fall asleep alone. Often the baby will go to sleep as you try to implement this idea and sometimes, he won't. On the opposite, if your baby doesn't settle down and fusses, you can rock, hug, or even pick him up and give him back the breast, bottle, or pacifier and either start over in a few minutes or for his next nap.

So, you see, you will help your baby slowly and lovingly learn how to fall asleep without your help during the first few months of life. And that you can do without crying (yours or his).

What About Thumb and Finger Sucking?

If your baby sucks her fingers unconscious, this is a completely different situation from using a bottle, pacifier or breast. If your baby has to find comfort in sucking her fingers, he/she learns to manage her own hands and doesn't always rely on someone else to support. Current opinions differ as to whether it is a good idea to let a baby get into this habit, but most experts agree that encouraging a young baby to suck their own fingers does not cause harm. As you might imagine, the biggest problem is that at any age some babies don't give up the habit, so you finally have to step in.

Waking for Night Feedings. Most pediatricians suggest that parents should not let an infant sleep without feeding for more than three or four hours, and the vast majority of babies wake up far more often than this. (Remember, too, that there are a handful of great babies that can go longer.) No matter what, the baby wakes up at night. The goal is to know when to pick her up for a night's meal, and when to let her go back to sleep alone.

This is a time when your instincts and intuition really need to be focused. That is when you should strive to learn how to read the signals from your infant. Here's a tip I'm surprised to never read in a baby book, but for you to learn it is critically important. Babies make plenty of sleeping noises, from grunts to whimpers to screaming outright, and those sounds don't always signify awakening. Those are what I call sleeping sounds, and during these episodes the baby is almost or even fully asleep. These are not the cry which means, "Mommy, I need you! "They're just sounds of night. I recall when my first daughter, Angela, slept in a cradle next to my bed as a child. Her cries had frightened me several times, yet she was asleep in my arms before I even had to sit down from cradle to rocking chair. She made noises in her sleep. In my attempt to respond to every cry of my daughter, I did, in fact, teach her to wake up more often! You need to listen carefully and watch your kid. Learn to distinguish between inactive sounds and hungry and awake sounds. If he/she's really up and hungry you're going to want to feed her as soon as possible. If you respond right away when he/she's tired, he/she'll most likely get back to sleep easily. But if you let her cry intensify, he/she's going to wake up more, and it's going to be harder and take longer for her to go back to sleep. Not to mention you'll be wide awake then, too! If your baby makes noises in the night, listen carefully; if he/she makes noises in the morning-let her sleep. If he/she's really waking up, be quick to tend to her.

For Breastfeeding or Co-Sleeping Mothers

It has become clear that a great many new mothers are spending some or all of their nights with their children. You'll probably synchronize your sleep cycles while you breastfeed and co-sleep with your infant. This means that both of you will undergo simultaneous midcycle awakenings. When this happens, it's a wonderful indication that you and your baby have found perfect harmony in sleep; and it will make your waking at night simpler, because when your baby wakes you won't be awakened from a deep sleeping state. It's easy for you to add your baby to your breast, in your partially awake state, and then, when your baby falls back to sleep quickly, so do you.

When you and your baby are in your brief periods of awakening during the night, he may just breathe noisily or move around, and you will automatically attach him to the breast; both of you will drift back to sleep. This is a beautiful, peaceful experience when you have a neonate lying next to you, and it can be the best solution for much-craved sleep for a new mother. Yet, a problem lies beneath the surface of that peaceful scenario. At every brief waking, your baby will come and expect a nurse. And if you recall Chapter 2, which outlined the basic facts of sleep, (you read that, right?) your baby has a brief awakening every hour or so throughout the night. While this arrangement may be appropriate to you for the early newborn months, it is a very unusual mother who will still love it 10 or 12 months later.

Sleeping Noises

The key is getting your co-sleeping baby to feel comfortable sleeping next to you without having to order Mommy's all-night snack bar every hour! Babies create a wide array of sleeping noises. Not all of these say, "I'm awake and want to feed." Learning how to pretend to be asleep while listening to Baby's sounds is the best long-term sleep enhancer for a co-sleeping baby. And wait. Without your help your baby may just fall back to sleep. If he/she needs breastfeeding, that you will know soon enough.

Help Your Baby Differentiate Day from Night

A newborn baby sleeps about sixteen to eighteen hours per day and this cycle is evenly distributed over six to seven brief periods of time. You will help your baby distinguish between nighttime and daytime sleep, and thus make him sleep longer during nighttime periods. Start by making your baby take his daytime naps in a lit room where he can hear the sounds of the day, maybe a bassinet or cradle located in your home's main area. Make dark and silent nightsleep. In the middle of the night, that means no talking, singing or lights. Use white noise to cover up family noises if your house is noisy during baby's bedtime. Light background music, a heater or a fan's hum (safety precautions taken), or any other steady sound can be white noise. You can even buy tiny clock radios with white-noise functions (they sound like spring rain or a babbling brook), or cassette tapes with calm sounds of nature or even womb sounds. You can also help your baby distinguish day naps from night sleep by using a nighttime bath and a pyjamas transition to show the difference between both. Keep your feedings still and mellow at night. In the middle of the night there's no need to talk or sing to your little one; leave all that for the daytime.

Nighttime Bottle-Feeding with Ease

If you are feeding your baby with bottles, make sure that everything you need for night feeding is close-up and ready to use. The goal is to keep the baby in a sleepy state and to nod to sleep right off. If you have to rush to the kitchen to make a bottle as baby fusses or cries, you'll only bring both of you to the point of being wide awake, and what may have been a brief waking at night will turn into a long wakefulness time.

Nighttime Slides

If your baby wakes in the night every hour or two, you don't have to change her diaper every time. Once, thinking back to when Angela was a child and I was a "new mom," when she woke up I dutifully changed her every hour or two. Sometimes I changed one dry diaper to another new one. Finally, I discovered that I was more "tuned in" than she was to the diaper problem! I suggest you put your baby in a good nighttime diaper, and do a quick check when he/she wakes. Switch her only if you need to, and do so in the dark as quickly and quietly as you can. When changing the infant, use a tiny nightlight and avoid any bright lights that may signify daytime. Have your changing supplies packed and near to Baby's bed, and make sure you clean the sleepy butt with a warm cloth. (Take a look at the many types of baby-wipe warmers available, and keep one near your changing station at night.)

Nighttime Cues

You'll want to create special cues for bedtime sleep. A regular, reliable routine at bedtime that begins at least thirty minutes before sleep is very helpful in getting baby to coordinate his sleep pattern day/night.

Don't let your baby sleep too long

Try not to let your child take a snack too long. If your little one sleeps a lot during the day, including a period of three to five hours, and then often gets up at night, he/she may have her days and nights mixed up. (Of course, there are those few babies that take long naps and then sleep well at night, but if your baby were like this you wouldn't read this book now, would you?) Sometimes it's a hard rule not to allow too long a nap. It's quick to "take advantage" of your baby's long nap to catch up when you're sleep-deprived, and you've fallen behind on your own chores and obligations. While this may be beneficial in the short run, it may conflict with nighttime sleep, making it more difficult for you to work during daytime. It also extends the time that your baby is sorting her sleep into short, daytime naps and long sleeping nights.

This is one of the times we're able to break the law of never waking a sleeping child. If your baby has napped for more than two or three hours, gently wake her up and allow her to stay awake and play for a while. Many children, like my second child, Vanessa, are such sleepy neonates that they cannot be wakened by an earthquake! We have a family portrait in her Daddy's arms with a sleeping four-week-old Vanessa as absolutely nothing would wake her up for the photo. Here are a couple of tips for waking such a sleepy baby when it's time to get up and eat:

- Try waking your baby during a lighter sleeping stage.
- Watch herarms, legs and face for movement. If the limbs of your baby dangle limply, he/she will be especially hard to wake up.
- Give the baby a change of diaper or rub a damp washcloth over his nose.
- Unwrap your baby and unwrap her (in a warm room) down to her diaper and T-shirt.
- Burp him into a seated position.
- Give Baby a rubbing back.
- Take off Baby's socks and rub her feet or wiggle her toes.
- Play "this little piggy."
- Move the arms and legs of Baby under a gentle routine of exercise.
- Prop infant seat baby in the center of family activity.
- Keep your child upright, and sing to her.

You may also be able to shorten these prolonged naps by setting him down in a room with daylight and a bit of noise for his nap and keeping night sleep very dark and quiet. Newborn babies do a lot of sleeping over the day. Yet, very soon, that will change. Understanding how to go about your usual daily life with a baby around can be a challenge, but it is important that you start treating your baby as a little person who keeps you company all day long. Don't assume you've got to save every job for the periods your baby sleeps. Start now to include your baby awake in your daily chores. Babies, after all, love to watch and learn and you are the most important teacher of your kid. He/she'll enjoy being part of your everyday life, and you'll also enjoy her company.

Watch for symptoms of tiredness

One way to encourage good sleep is to get acquainted with the sleepy signs of your baby and put her down to sleep as soon as he/she is tired. A baby can't sleep, nor can he/she comprehend her own sleepy signs. Yet it is usually unhappy to have a baby who is encouraged to stay awake while her body craves sleep. Over time, this pattern evolves into sleep deprivation, further complicating the growth of your baby's sleep maturity.

Most newborns can handle wakefulness in only about two hours. When Baby gets overtired, he becomes over-stimulated and finds it more difficult to fall asleep and stay asleep. Wait for the moment of magic when Baby is tired, but not overtired. These are some of the signs that your baby may show you— he may show you just one or two; you'll get to know your baby over time;

- A lull in movement and activity
- Quiet down
- Losing interest in people and toys (looking away)
- Looking "glazed"
- Fussing

- Rubbing eyes
- Yawning

Learn to read the sleepy signs of your baby and put him to bed when that window of opportunity presents itself.

Keep your baby relaxed

Babies are as different as we adults are from each other, and over time you can learn to understand your own baby. Here are a couple of ideas to make kids comfortable. Experiment with them, and you'll soon find out which ones are best for your little one. Swaddling babies arrive fresh from an environment (the womb) where they've been held tightly. Some babies are most comforted by wrapping them securely in a receiving blanket, when parents create a womb-like setting for sleep. Your doctor, a veteran parent, or a baby book will give you step-by-step instructions on how to swaddle your infant. If your baby likes swaddling, you may want to use it to help her to sleep longer at night. Ask your doctor if your baby can be securely swaddled in a blanket, too. When Baby starts moving around, this is not a safe way for her to sleep, as he/she can remove the blanket and get tangled. Another caution: If the air is dry, don't swaddle a baby; it can cause overheating, which is one of SIDS ' risk factors.

Cozy Cradle

Lots of new babies just get lost in a big crib. The baby can find that he/she likes a smaller cradle or bassinet. Most babies even scooter up to the cradle corner to wedge their head into the crevice— just as they were wedged in your pelvis. Make sure that when your baby is sleeping, if your cradle will rock, you lock it in a stationary position, and that it cannot be tipped over as he/she does this ritual of creeping into the corner.

Build a Nest

Because they've spent nine months curling into a tight ball, some new babies aren't comfortable lying flat on a firm mattress on their back. Nonetheless, the most important defense against SIDS is the back-sleeping on a firm mattress. An option that seems to keep many babies comfortable and help them sleep longer is to place them in a car seat, infant seat or stroller to sleep, keeping them in a curled position. This could help those babies who only sleep well while being cradled in the arms of Mommy or Daddy, or snugly curled into a sling. It offers a gentle approach for teaching Baby how to sleep out of your belly. If you use this idea, safety rules meanyou mustkeep your baby in sight. However, if your baby sleeps in a car seat or baby seat, make sure that he does not lean over with his head downwards. This can lead to trouble breathing. Help your baby keep his head up with specially made car-seat padding which provides extra support. A potential drawback to this theory is that your baby may become used to sleeping upright, which may cause problems later when trying to lie down sleeping. Therefore car-seat naps should be interspersed with lying on a flat surface.

Sweet Sounds

A number of companies are now making recordings of heartbeats that mimic what your baby heard in the womb. A new baby can be confident with these sounds. As already mentioned, quiet music or white noise can also work well.

Better Smells

A baby has a stronger sense of smell than an adult. Research shows that her scent helps a baby identify his own mother. You can tuck it in your shirt for a few hours if you have a small, healthy stuffed animal or baby blanket, and then put it in the cradle while the baby sleeps, following all the safety precautions.

Warm Bed

It can be jarred awake when a sleeping baby is placed on cold sheets. You can warm up her sleeping spot with a wrapped hot water bottle or a heating pad set on low while you are feeding your baby. Remove the warmer from the crib before you lay down your infant, and always run your arm through the whole area to make sure it isn't too hot. One option is using flannel crib sheets instead of the warmer cotton sheets.

Make Yourself Comfortable

I still have to hear a parent tell me he/she or he wants to get up all night in order to take care of the needs of an infant. As much as we love our little packages, when you wake up again and again, night after night, it is difficult. Because it's a reality your baby is going to wake you up, you can be as confident as you can.

Consider Night Waking

With your newborn baby the first step is to learn to relax right now about night waking. Feeling nervous or upset about waking up isn't going to change a thing. It is much like a fourth stage of labor— a very, very short period of time in your life, and you will probably not be able to easily remember the debilitating tiredness later on. The situation will improve day by day; and before you know it, your little baby will no longer be so little— he/she'll walk and talk and get into everything in sight during the day and sleep peacefully throughout the night. But you are now in this new-born–no-sleep period, so do what you can to get through it as safely as you can. Here are a few suggestions for making your nightlife less stressful for yourself:

- Make your nightlife place as cozy and comfortable as possible. If you are feeding your baby while sitting in a chair, I suggest you move the most comfortable chair into Baby's room for the moment. When using a rocking chair, ensure that it has soft padding on the front and back. Get a soft footstool and put a table next to you for your water glass, a book, a night light, and anything else that makes these night episodes more welcoming.
- Make sure everything you need is ready and waiting for you to bottle-feed. (Wonderful portable bottle stations are available. Check out the Dusk to Dawn Bottle Warmer at

onestepahead.com as one choice I've been told is convenient.)

- Invest in a specially designed breastfeeding pillow or play with how to use bed and sofa pillows to help both the baby and you during your feeding sessions.
- Make sure you're really happy with breastfeeding in bed. Many mothers lament a sore back from bedtime nursing. Generally, this is from arching your back to bringing your breast to your infant. Instead, let your baby fold around you in a comfortable and restful position. Babies are incredibly versatile and will fasten into any space you require. Even a broad eighteen-month-old will comfortably curl himself into the space if you lie on your side and get your knees up.

When you and your baby are co-sleeping, make sure that the bed is large enough to make you feel comfortable. If you are squashed, invest in a bigger mattress or in a second one.

- During these early months, plan your life for your baby as much as possible. Stop scheduling events at night that mess with your bedtime routine or keepyou out too late. The world is going to wait several months.
- Relax, and go slow. It's a very brief period in your life. Stop doing all those things that are less important in favor of the most important: taking care of your new child. It's OK— truly.

Fill Baby's Tummy Before Sleep

Try to make the last feeding before bedtime a complete one. If baby nods off after feeding from one breast or after taking half a bottle, shift her around, untuck the blanket, tickle those toes, and encourage her to finish the feeding; otherwise, he/she may wake up very soon to "finish" her feeding.

Create Restful Feeding Sessions

One piece of advice you'll hear from time to time is "sleep when baby sleeps during the day." Nice idea, but as a working mom, the last thing I can do is sleep while baby sleeps! And I'm prepared to bet that your days are as full as mine. Therefore, long, blissful naps seem to be out of the question. But, you can rest during the day while feeding your baby. During those first few months, your baby will eat regularly. Relaxing and feeding your baby is your work. Don't sit there and be nervous about all the things you should be doing. This is what you should do in your baby's life during these first few months. Each time you sit to feed your new baby, follow these steps:

- Relax
- Breathe slowly
- Push down your shoulders, and then relax. (Mothers tend to raise their shoulders during feeding, particularly in the first few months. If your shoulders are raised somewhere around your face, this causes muscle tension in your back, shoulders and neck.)
- Shake your head to work out stress.

- Take advantage of this opportunity to look at your beautiful little one for a few minutes of happy baby time. Come to make memories.
- Write, if you like. (Or read to your baby.)
- Watch TV or a movie, or listen to music, if you relax.

Simplify your life

In these early months of your baby's life, simplify your life as much as you can. Relax the standards regarding housekeeping. Graciously accept whatever support somebody offers you. (Repeat after me: "Sure, thank you, it would be nice.") Your first priority is to take care of your new baby right now.

Have Realistic Expectations

The newborn child is not going to sleep through the night. There are no easy approaches to sleep competence, and no shortcuts. When you focus on your need for a full night's sleep, you can simply push yourself to the point of crying over what you can't have right now. The best advice I can give you is to know that your baby's going to pass quickly with these early months. And then you'll look back on those memories of holding your baby in your arms with fondness.

Solutions for Older Babies— Four Months to Two Years

You have to work out where the problem lies. Is it in the routine of your baby, in their management of it, or simply in others' minds? If you can honestly say that you want to change your baby's sleeping habits because they disturb you and your family personally, then you're ready to read on.

Get Your Baby Ready

Fill That Daytime Tummy

Make sure your baby gets enough to eat during the day, especially if he's only breastfed or fed formula. Many babies get into the habit of breastfeeding or drinking bottles throughout the night, taking up then an unfair amount of their daily calories. Some babies need to tip the feeding scales back towards the daytime to sleep longer at night. Ensure that the majority of food options are safe for those little ones eating solids. Yeah, your kid loves cheese and that's the only thing he/she'll eat, however good nutrition rules say he/she can have more variety. For overall health good nutrition is critical, including good sleep. Check what the child is eating in the hours before bedtime. Munching on foods conducive to good sleep?

Many foods are easier to digest than others, and are less likely to interfere with sleep cycles. Think about "comfort food"— complex, healthy carbohydrates and nutritious proteins. There are countless choices: whole-grain cereals (easy on the sugar!), oatmeal, brown rice, yogurt, milk, meats left over. Sweet cravings are fulfilled by vegetables and frozen peas (for older children who will not chokeon them). In comparison, a lot of foods seem to "power" the body a little bit. Search for secret caffeine, as well as other stimulants. While current scientific wisdom suggests that sugar does not cause children to behave hyperactively, I also suspect an effect on the ability and willingness to calm down and fall asleep. Sugar and chocolate cake cookies are simply not good options for late in the day. If your kid goes on food jags like most, take heart. Note that, rather than a day, pediatricians look at a child's diet from a week's perspective. In other words, when measuring the healthiness of your child's diet, consider proportions of the major food groups eaten over the course of a whole week.

Breastfeed More During the Day

If your baby is used to regular night feedings, during those long, relaxed feeding sessions, he/she takes in a good portion of her calories. During the day, you may need to nurse more often for a while in order to compensate for the nighttime feedings he/she may give up. Your growing baby wakes up every night for the warmth and emotional connection as much as for milk— especially if you're busy working or tending to other kids during the day. You should give your little one extra cuddles and extra breastfeeding during the day if you are prone to this, to help her adapt to giving up those overnight nursing sessions. Pay attention to the types of food you consume, as it may affect breast milk. Check for the reaction of your baby when you drink coffee, tea, or cola or when you have dairy, nuts, or gaseous foods like broccoli, beans, and cauliflower. As in the case of little Austen, your curious, busy kid may be too involved to pause for eating or even for nursing during the day. In this scenario, consider delivering "food on the go" to your lively baby— finger food he/she can bring with her. Another choice is giving her food bites as he/she plays. The goal is to help her get the calories of her full day into the daytime and the nighttime.

Check Baby's Nighttime Comfort

Make sure the bed is very comfortable for children. Dress him up according to room temperature, making sure he's neither too cold nor too hot. Buy thick blanket sleeping pajamas or baby-bag sleepers if your home is cool at night and put on a T-shirt (the full-body type that snaps at the crotch.) If the season is hot, cool the room with an open window or fan, but follow all the safety rules if you do so.

CHAPTER 11: STAYING IN THE (HABIT) LOOP

If you have followed the plan outlined in this book there are two possible outcomes.

The first, most likely outcome, is that your child sleeps much better in the evening. I assume that you, too, are. Enjoy the fruits of your labor and the satisfaction of feeling like a normal human again. If that's the case, there are a couple of steps to ensure your child continues to sleep well — and to make sure you don't panic at the first sign of trouble.

The second possible scenario is that things still don't go according to plan. I'll look at some common problems, including bedtime issues, nighttime awakenings, and how to cope with the dreaded early morning wake-up calls.

Locking in High-Quality Sleep: How to Maintain

If things went well at this stage, you're probably pretty anxious. You may have experienced a night or two of blissful, uninterrupted sleep in the past, only for weeks or months to have the old patterns reassert themselves. I assure you that this time is different because you used the pattern loop to form the actions of your infant. There are a couple of things you need to do to lock in and make these patterns effortless. How to ride a bike is like how? You have to think about every step when you start and one bad fall will shake your confidence. Over time, the ride is seamless and without struggling to stay upright, you can enjoy your ride.

Note, to become formed and automatic, habits take about a month. This is true for you and your child alike. Good sleeping habits are actually two sets of interlocking habits— yours and the one of your children. So, if you've finally gotten good sleep, celebrate your hard work, but just don't relax.

Next, you have a month to be consistent. I don't mean a month from the time you started— I mean a month from the time your child's sleep got better. I recommend avoiding holidays, family visits or any other significant changes to your routine during this period, if at all possible. Having a babysitter so you can go out for a night is OK if you believe it won't disrupt your child's routine. (Generally, most children behave better for their babysitters than for their parents— parental care is a much more desirable consequence than babysitting attention. However, I remember a babysitter who didn't put my son to bed because he didn't want to go. Needless to say, after a nice night out, my wife and I weren't excited about having to go to bed. It means keeping the same regular bedtime and bedtime routine when you're staying in a hotel, but this can be complicated if you share a room after having your child sleep separately. This is an imperfect solution, and may result in a temporary setback; I will explain how to deal with this later.

You should relax a bit but not completely after the first regular month of high-quality sleep. After that, it's okay to allow variety on one or two nights a week, such as going out to dinner at the house of another family or a movie outing. Recognize that this may result in a minor disturbance to sleep, but stay confident in the program you have set up.

The last thing to remember is not to panic if you're having a bad evening or two. This is happening toeveryone, and can probably be predicted at some point.

When to Expect Trouble and How to Troubleshoot

As a teacher, I have often felt the sense of fear that arises when a previously solved question returns. (Like the time we walked deep in the woods and my then four-year-old was swarming with bugs and pooping his pants. You're not going to be psyched, but you need to calm down and stop panicking, and I'm not just telling you this for your mental health. Remember, any attention you offer to behavior— positive or negative— you're not going to just reinforce the behavior.

Sleep Regression

Here's a secret — when your pediatrician says, "Your child is going through a phase," he/she means, "Your child is doing something mysterious and annoying and I hope it's going to pass soon, because I'm not sure what to do about it." This is widely used to refer to bouts of sleep disruption that seem to come out of nowhere in children who have been sleeping well — the dreaded sleep regression.

I don't like the word "sleep regression." It's a concept that has gained a lot of traction in parenting circles and with sleep consultants— a sleep coach named Rob Lindeman did some legwork and noticed that this phrase began to popularize around 2008, according to Google search data— but it doesn't suit any actual physiological change in children's sleep. What the parents typically mean when using this word is an unwanted or unexplained disturbance in the sleep of their infant. Most parents undergo one when their children develop an understanding of object permanence around the age of four to six months; the child has a normal biological awakening at night and begins to recognize that there is no mom or dad and begins to weep.

As it turns out, interruption of sleep is often correlated with new developmental accomplishments. As Dr. Danny Lewin, a Children's National Health System sleep specialist says of sleep regression, "Do not see it as a loss or an issue, see it as a warning. Developmentally, there is something going on that is a positive, evolving improvement in their growth in most common cases. "It's hard to know exactly how this happens in pre-verbal children. I am always fascinated by the relation between pre-verbal children's milestones and sleep disruption. I sometimes wonder if kids are so nervous about these milestones that when they wake up in the night, they want to play. Or maybe they're tired, and sore.

Common developmental attainments associated with sleep disruption include:

The concurrent evolution of crawling, the notion of object permanence, and stranger anxiety (6–9 months),learning to walk (12–15 months), potty training (2–4 years),understanding narrative in TV shows and movies (6–8 years)—when children can better understand cause and effect (for example, in stories with "good guys" and "bad guys"), it can be associated with more anxiety, which often flares up.

One thing you need to look at if your child starts experiencing a sleep disturbance is the media to which your child is subjected. My boys are three years apart in age, and the younger one is more interested in fun shows and video games of his big brother than in content more appropriate for maturity. And, at age six, he ended up watching Ghostbusters. It didn't really scare him but for that age, frankly, it's not fitting. Even age-appropriate media can sometimes have photos that resonate with your child negatively and really scare him. After seeing some freaky swamp monsters on the TV cartoon Super Friends, I remember having problems sleeping. However, this is nothing compared to the nighttime fear I had after seeing the commercial for The Day After — a film involving a nuclear attack on the U.S.— at age 10. I hoped in a frenzyfor months every night that there would be no nuclear war that night. If your older child struggles, ask him if he is afraid of anything.

Minor Illnesses

Illnesses are less predictable but can be equally disruptive aschanges in development. These most often take the form of viruses — like common cold, ear infections, or bugs in the stomach. These may also be due to outbreaks of underlying issues— worsening eczema itching, coughing and wheezing in an asthma infant, or even plain old constipation. Do your best to keep your routine in the throes of your child's sickness, but don't get frustrated when your child needs you during the night. Luckily, when the illness gets better, the associated sleep disruptions tend to go away provided you go back to your routine.

Vacations

Remember when you and your partner enjoyed long, late meals with a couple of drinks, sleeping the next day, and then relaxing on the beach? No, me either.

If you haven't worked it out yet, holidays with young children can be fun but they're not restful. If you interrupt your normal routine, you begin to appreciate how importantstructure is to the actions of your child. You may be living with other families who have various bedtime routines and rules. You're likely sharing your child's room. You may be consuming different foods, and may have more face time than usual for you and your infant, which may result in nerves becoming frayed. And I can guarantee you won't sleep unless your partner or other family member whisks away your kids at the crack of dawn.

Here are some details I've learned about optimizing sleep in our adventures:

- Honor the routine. When we go on holiday, we're always trying hard to maintain the sleep times of our babies. This was more complicated when they were napping. For special occasions such as weddings, festivals, or movies, we bend the rules of course. Some "sneaky night" may also be necessary, as the kids get pretty tucked away.

- Recognize that different rules apply to other communities, and be flexible. My children also point to me when other families who we are with have different rules (usually if the children have more iPad time than mine). That can be very difficult when some kids go later to bed or get up earlier than your kids. Make sure your kids know that they may have different rules for their peers or siblings, and it's OK. Encourage your kids to be versatile and consider certain social variations. Adults can assist with that process as well. I really appreciate that when we are together, my sister-in-law, who gives her children more screen time than we do with ours, encourages her children to abide by our rules, so that everyone can play.

What to Do If You Are Still Having Trouble

Often, you may be having some residual problems despite your best efforts. If you have followed the strategies in this book but are still struggling after a couple of weeks, I suggest that you start with your bedtime cue but maybe pause with consequences until you can find out what is not working.

Next, look again for medical issues which might influence the sleep of your child by making an appointment with your pediatrician. There are common problems that may interrupt nighttime sleep. Checking for a condition like obstructive sleep apnea might even be worth considering an overnight sleep check.

Paying close attention to bedtime and the habit process will resolve certain persistent issues. A small adjustment can sometimes bring big results. Here are some of the most commonly used approaches to seek if your child still has a hard time.

Go to bed early. We were on holiday with cousins and all the children got up earlier than usual. If you want to catch up on your sleep, the best chance is to go to bed.

Make the room somber. Close the curtains. If you need to, don't hesitate to hang towels over the windows; that can help your children sleep a little longer in the morning. You can drape a towel or blanket over a Pack' n Play for children over a year, carry KidCo Peapod travel beds for babies, or try a Dream Tent (available for older children at www.mydreamtents.com).

- It is critical that you mask sound. We usually bring our sound machines, but for white noise or nature sounds (I use the Nature space app) you can also run a fan or use an app on your phone.
- The sleep arrangements are creative. Some years ago, we were staying at a vacation home with several relatives. For

kids used to getting their own room, sharing rooms can be a bit tricky; older kids should be advised to let others sleep when they wake up early. We may be a little chatty at bedtime too, but that's part of the fun. One of the difficulties may be the need for shared beds, particularly if you've just weaned your child out of this environment. I advise you to put your child in a Pack' n Play (adhering to safe sleep standards of course) or on an air mattress for older children. If you end up having to share a bed with your kids, carefully explain that this is a special sleepover and that the rules are different from those at home. When you get home, you may get a little pushback but stick to your signs and implications and your routine will return to normal quickly.

- Jet lag can be difficult. Jet lag happens as you fly east or west across time zones, as your body clock is out of clock time process. You can plan aheada little by putting your kids to bed a few days later before they head west or waking them up a little earlier before they travel east. The key effect, when traveling west, can be a really early bedtime and wake time, or vice versa when traveling east. Once children are exposed to natural light they begin to adapt quickly. When possible stop "sneaky night," and seek to get to the "right" bedtime as soon as possible (according to the clock). An option to having your home time zone schedule may be for short trips.

- Don't think about this teddy bear. That one is very self-explanatory. Don't miss it at home. Don't forget to rent it in the car, at the airport, or at the diner. Trust me— I was burnt before.

Problems with Falling Asleep

Try a later bedtime

If your child still fails to fall asleep at night, revisiting your child's bedtime might be worthwhile— specifically when turning the lights out. Look back to your last two or three days' sleep diaries and look at when your child actually falls asleep. So switch the lights-out time of your child to the moment when he actually falls asleep. Here's the key — keep his wake-time constant. When he falls asleep within 15 to 20 minutes, push his bedtime earlier every few nights by ten minutes until you get back to 8:30 p.m. And, earlier. For more information on that process, it's called "bedtime fading."

ARCH for hidden effects

Take a careful look at any inadvertent effects that you or others are having at home. It seems generally to be a lack of consistency. Here are a few questions you can ask yourself:

1. Do bedtime and nap time always happen at the same time?
2. Is it the same bedtime routine every night?
3. Are you regularly listening to your child in the way you intended?

Does everybody who cares for your child (you, your mom, grandma, the sitter) do the same things at bedtime and at night? Work to eliminate any inconsistencies you might find.

CHAPTER 12: BABY'S SLEEPING (FINALLY!) BUT MOMMY'S NOT

Your baby is finally sleeping after adopting the either the cry it outor No-Cry Sleep Solution-making your sleep schedule, charting your success, persevering night after night. It is incredible. It's marvelous. Everything is fine with your house's sandman. Your child sleeps through the night. But you don't.

What's Happening?

A couple of things have disturbed your sleep in the past year or more. Issues such as pregnancy, accompanied by a baby, and maybe followed by another pregnancy, and one or more children. If your baby entered your family by adoption, throughout the long and involved process, and then through the early months of baby sleeplessness, you have lost sleep. You may not know that you got into the habit of getting up during the night.

An average night's sleep requires multiple night wakings and a body that has become accustomed to some degree of isolation from sleep. It's definitely been a long time since you truly had the sleep of a full night. Of course, far longer than you know! In reality, many parents forget what their sleep patterns were like before children came into their lives. Most believe they used to regularly and without interruption earn eight hours. For most adults, eight hours is the amount of time recommended by sleep experts. In fact, though, adults sleep an average of about seven hours per night according to the National Sleep Foundation. In fact, at least half of all adults have trouble sleeping — sleeping and staying asleep — kid or no baby.

In other words, if you weren't sleeping like a log before baby, you're not going to sleep like a log now either. Your present sleep condition has yet another thing to remember. When we age (and you have done that over the past couple of years, you know), the amount of sleep we need and the amount of sleep we get continues to decrease, and sometimes the sleep problems are that. The effect of the ebb and flow of monthly hormones on our sleep has also been acknowledged by recent studies by the National Sleep Foundation.

How to Get a Good Night's Sleep?

Because you've just undergone a time of regular night waking, I don't have to warn you that your whole life can be affected by the quality and amount of your sleep. For your health and well-being, getting adequate, restful sleep is essential. Everyone has different sleep needs, and according to your own health you should calculate your sleep requirements. Let your body tell you what it wants, and make every effort to listen to it. Learn to recognize the signs you're sleeping well or not having enough. The following are some useful tips for optimizing adult sleep that I have come across for this book in my comprehensive research. Check the list and use as many as you want. It should be beneficial to add even one or two of these suggestions. This is an important point to keep in mind. Often people who have been deprived of sleep for any length of time actually feel more difficult when they start making changes to improve their patterns of sleep. The good news is that this is short-lived and you'll feel better emotionally and physically as soon as you adapt to your improved sleep.

Review the suggestions below, try out those that apply to you, and build your own sleep schedule. You will soon be asleep— like a newborn (a baby that doesn't wake up every two hours).

Stop Worrying about sleep Now

It's great your baby is sleeping better. That was the target when you purchased this book and you were already successful. Once you sleep better, it's just a matter of time as well— once you're accustomed to the new routine of your son, and you're sure he is too. The cruel irony is that you're thinking about lying in bed because you can't fall or stay asleep. So, please relax. Ignore these instructions, and come to sleep. Turn your clock off and don't think about whether or not you're asleep. Through fretting about it you cannot force yourself to sleep. The best you can do is to set up good sleeping patterns and pursue them through the night. As a busy parent, the dilemma may be exacerbated by worrying that your sleep time willtake up valuable time that could be spent doing other things. You either get to bed far too late, or you lie in bed and feel guilty about it, worrying about all the other things you "should" do. Give permission to lie down. You need it for your body, it's necessary for your health, and it's good for your soul. Remember that if you're well-fed, your baby will also benefit because you're going to be a happier mum (or daddy). And if you breastfeed or are pregnant your improved sleep willhelp both you and your infant.

Pay Off Your Sleep Debt

We build a sleep debt with each additional sleepless night when we don't get enough sleep. If you still feel deprived of sleep, try to collect as many more minutes of sleep as you can. Set aside some extra sleep for two weeks to squeeze it in. Make it a precedent. Go to bed early whenever you can, sleep a few minutes later, take a nap if you can. Even an extra sleeping hour will help you pay off at least a portion of your sleep debt. You should feel much better and be able to move on to developing a healthy routine for sleep. When you really cannot find extra time for sleep, then ignore this concept and work on developing a healthy routine for sleep. You may find that dissipating your sleep debt will take a month or twoof working on your new sleep schedule, but it will. Once you've developed your own plan, you'll find that sleep isn't on your list of things to think about anymore. Instead, it'll only be an easy, normal part of your life, the way it's for your kids.

Set Your Body Clock

Your body has an internal alarm clock for sleep time and awake time. The clock is set by the continuity of your sleep schedule, which makes it work for you. If your bedtime and awake time are different every day, it undermines the effectiveness of this amazing nature gift; your clock is out of sync. At inappropriate times, you will find yourself exhausted or worried, sometimes feeling as if you could fall asleep standing up during the day, but then lying wide awake in bed at night... It explains why on Monday morning a lot of people have trouble waking up. If you have a specific wake and sleep time during the week, you'll probably find that you're waking up just before your alarm goes off by Friday morning, and it's difficult to stay awake during the late-night movie on Friday night. Come Monday morning, when the morning alarm goes off, you're groggy and tired. What's happened is that your biological clock took control by the end of the week due to your regular wake-sleep schedule. Yet come over the weekend youmovedyour bedtime later, and if you're lucky enough to do it, you'll even sleep late in the morning. It basically cancels the setting on our clocks and we must start all over again by Monday.

The mismatch is a simple one to fix — and the handy tool that will do the trick is a good, consistent sleep schedule. Choose a specific bedtime and wake-up time; stick to it as close as possible, seven days a week. Clearly, occasionally your busy life will change the routine. Once in a while you will deviate from your strategy without doing too much to get things upset. But ultimately, if you stick as faithfully as possible to your routine, your sleep will be more relaxing, and you'll be healthier and more alert. Your body clock willfunction as it should, helping you to tick productively through your day and to wind down peacefully at night. Of course, with a varying sleep schedule, a few lucky people can work well, but they are the exception. This simple, powerful advice is helping most people immensely.

Get Organized

Your stress level increases when your days are hectic and disorganized; the normal physiological and emotional responses to this stress hamper your ability to sleep. So by getting at the root of it, we can combat this kind of sleeplessnessbybecoming more focused and purposeful during the day. A set daily schedule or to-do list will make you feel more in control of your days. You'll be able to relax a little with the countless critical details of each day written down. Think of it as getting out of your mind and onto paper all the dates and times and jobs, freeing up a little breathing room upstairs. And you're not going to wonder late at night, "What do I need to do? What was it I forgot?"In your lists and on your schedule, it's all right. Keep a pad and a pencil next to your bed should an important idea or mission pop into your mind as you begin to drift off. Write it downandlet it go.

Avoid Caffeine Late in the Day

Caffeine remains from six to fourteen hours in your bloodstream! Around midnight and beyond, the caffeine in that after-dinner cup of coffee still sticks around in your system. Caffeine contains a chemical that induces wakefulness and hyperactivity, which is why many people find their morning coffee so relaxing. Caffeine tolerance levels differ, so you'll have to deal with how much you can drink and how late you can drink it without disturbing your sleep. If you're a nursing mother, look carefully at your baby to see if caffeine is impacting her too. While no research has established the link between caffeine and the sleeplessness of an infant, we do know that diet affects breast milk consistency, quantity, and palatability, so a correlation isn't entirely farfetched. (Many of the breastfeeding mothers mentioned a perceived an effect of caffeine on their infant, so it's worth looking at your own situation.) Keep in mind that caffeine is more than just a coffee ingredient. It includes tea (green as well as black), cola, some other soft drinks (including root beer and orange - check the labels), chocolate, even some over-the-counter painkillers, albeit in smaller quantities. Better choices are warm milk or herbal teas for pre-bed drinks, which will carry the relaxed state required for sleep.

Look Out for Drug and Alcohol Effects

If you take any drug, ask your doctor or pharmacist if there are any side effects to it. We always know what drugs make us drowsy, but we don't understand some of them have the opposite effect — acting as a stimulant. Likewise, one or two evening glasses of wine or beer will not necessarily affect sleep, and could carry it on. But more than that can have a rebound effect, triggering an episode of insomnia in the middle of the night, a few hours later. Alcohol can also disturb the consistency of your sleep, making it superficial and disturbing regular cycles of dreams.

Consider exercise a part of your day

There are many advantages of balancing your day with regular exercise and better sleep is at the top of the list. Several studies have shown that mild, regular exercise decreases insomnia and improves the quality of sleep (not to mention normal, everyday experience). The trick to using exercise to improve sleep is to follow a regular pattern: moderate aerobic exercise of thirty to forty-five minutes, three to four days a week. Make sure to finish the exercise at least three hours before bedtime for best results; exercise leaves most people too energized to sleep immediately afterward. (There are variations though. Somepeople find that strenuous exercise makes them fall asleep easily afterward. Try to find out if this applies to you.) You may think your baby precludes you from going out and exercising. Quite the opposite! Your baby is supplying you with the perfect excuse for a daily walk behind the stroller. If the weather gets in your way in winter, head for an indoor shopping mall with room to roam. This may not work for you every day, and you may have to leave your wallet at home, but it's an effective way for many parents to squeeze in a walk. Nevertheless, most babies love it and benefit from the stimulation (which can actually help baby sleep too).

Here are a few more ways to integrate daily exercise into your life: When you work at home, use a treadmill, a stationary bike, or other gym equipment after you put your little one down for a nap.

- Jog the escalators up and down.
- Take your baby out, and do some gardening.

- When you work outside the homeclimb up and down the stairs at lunchtime or during a break, or take a walk around the block.
- Create a schedule to make the most of a gym or training space for employees.
- Walk regularly to the copy machine, mailroom, or toilet.
- Ideas for all:
- Play a video exercise and practice with your kid.
- Put some great music on and dance with your kids.
- Look for little ways to add exercise to your day, such as parking farther from the shop, using the stairs instead of the elevator, walking instead of driving to a local destination, going to school with your older children or playing outdoors with your children.
- Schedule family activities requiring movement and motion, such as biking, cycling, or beach or park breaks.

Make Your Environment Favorable to Sleep

Look at your bedroom well and make sure it's conducive to relaxing and a safe sleep. Each person is different but you need to review a checklist here.

- Rest assured. Are you comfortable with your mattress? Does it offer the amount of support you need? Do you like your blanket or comforter, or is it a source of nighttime aggravation? Is it the perfect softness and thickness for your pillow? Did you find the content relaxing and cozy? Do what you can to make the specifics better.

- Tempering. You wake often if you are too cold or too hot during sleep. Experiment until the optimum temperature has been reached. Find a way to please both of you if your partner has different preferences by adjusting the type of pajamas you wear, using a fan, or piling on extra blankets.
- Noise. With perfect silence, some people sleep better, while others prefer background music or white noise. Also, if one sleeping partner likes noise, but the other needs quiet, experiment,try earplugs or a personal music or sound headset.

Lighting. If in complete darkness you sleep easier, close your door. Open the blinds, or use a nightlight, if you like light. (Be cautious when using lights at night when you get up to use the bathroom or tend your baby. Bright light will trick your biological clock into believing its morning. Rely on low-wattage nightlights.) Again, if your partner likes open blinds and you like shutting them, decide whoseneeds are greater or find a compromise. You could buy a soft eye mask made just for that reason, or leave the blinds open on one side of the room, closed on the other — facing the closed window you'll feel darker.

Have your own bedtime routine.To help your baby sleep better, you may have introduced a bedtime routine. That same idea, too, will work for you. We parents often have a very comfortable routine to put our kids to bed.

After that soothing hour, when we've just fallen to sleep reading the story of bedtime, we run into high gear and sprint all over the house to do all those tasks that await our attention before we look up and— oh no! It is around midnight! Your own routine before bedtime will greatly enhance your ability to fall asleep and stay asleep. It can include something soothing, including reading, listening to music, or sitting with your partner sipping a cup of tea and chatting. Avoid having your mind or body activated in the hour before bed. Tasks such as responding to your e-mail, doing heavy home cleaning, or watching TV will keep you awake long after you're done. Try to keep the lights dim in the hour before bed if possible, as bright light strongly signals the body to jump into daytime action. Dim lighting and relaxing sounds help you get ready for a good night's sleep.

Eat Right and Eat Light Before Sleep.

You'll sleep better with neither too full nor too empty a stomach. A big meal will make you feel exhausted, but it will keep your body digesting, disrupting your sleep. An empty stomach will keepyou pained with hunger. It is usually best to have a happy medium. Have a light snack before bedtime, about an hour or two. Avoid gaseous, salty, sucrose, or spicy foods. Milk, bacon, cottage cheese, turkey, and cashews are some foods that have been found to help people sleep better. Experiment with figuring out which solutions are right for you.

Encourage relaxation and the onset of sleep. Even when we are lying in bed waiting for sleep, our mind and body are ready to act. The wheels turn and our minds keep us up. Focusing your mind on calm, calming thoughts is a helpful way of bringing sleep. Here are a few ways to do this:

- Repeat a common meditation or prayer to liberate the mind from daily activities and make it sleep-prime. Yoga stretches will help the muscles relax.

- Focus on breathing when repeating the word relax in a slow rhythm that is related to the exhales. And imagine that your breath passes in and out along with a beach wave.

- Use radical relaxation to encourage all body parts to relax. Start at the bottom. Feel the weight of your feet, get them to go limp and relax, and then imagine they've got a soft air flowing over them. Then move your right leg upwards, repeat the process. Go on to your left leg, and keep going up to your shoulders. (Most people are asleep or almost asleep when they get that far!) Maybe you want to incorporate some of the relaxation exercises you've learned in birth classes.

When engorgement is the issue, there is often a period of adjustment when a breastfed baby begins sleeping through the night. It's hard to believe, but your breasts are going to develop their own set of clocks. Diminished production during the night is quite common, and your milk production pattern will mirror your baby's new feeding pattern within a week of new sleep patterns. Your breasts are still constantly producing milk, so if your baby wakes to feed once in a while he will find enough for comfort there. Interestingly enough, if your baby suddenly starts to wake up again due to the spurts of teething, disease, or development, your milk production will change along with its needs (as long as you are feeding on demand). What a beautiful breastfeeding blessing!

Transition Time Strategies. Here are a few tips to make the adjustment period pass.

- Give your child a full feeding on both sides before bedtime and in the morning.
- Sleep with nursing pads or washcloths tucked inside your roomiest bra.
- Wake engorged, add a small number of warm compresses and pump (either by hand or with a breast pump). Don't pump a full feed because you are trying to trick your body into thinking the baby really wants the night feeding. Just release enough to keep yourself relaxed.
- Massage your breasts under the spray of water and take a warm shower. Maybe you'd like to lean forward so gravity will help you move some milk. This can help release enough milk to make you feel comfortable before your baby wakes up to nurse.
- Apply the breasts with a cold compress, or use ibuprofen to relieve pain or discomfort.
- If you're in pain and can't pump, go ahead and pick up your baby and put him on your breast. During their sleep, most infants will eat, and yours can suck enough to help you get back to sleep. Even if your baby wakes during this feeding, during the nursing session, he will fall straight back to sleep quickly.

- Be prepared for a little extra daytime feeding. Some babies that suddenly start to sleep longer at night will compensate for the lost feedings by nursing more during the day.
- If you have had plugged ducts or breast infections in the past, avoid repeating them by pumping or nursing your child enough to soften your breasts. Just try to minimize this so you can work out your schedule for the nighttime feeding. Remember your body must change the output to suit the new sleep schedule for your infant.
- Don't breastfeed! Your breasts still need to be cleaned, and this painful state will be improved by daily daytime feeding.

Pay attention to your own well-being, be careful when you have chronic insomnia or other serious sleep problems, or other health issues. See your physician as soon as possible.

Optimize your bedroom environment

Many people believe the environment of the bedroom and its setup are key factors for getting a good night's sleep. These factors include temperature, noise, exterior lights, and arrangement of the furniture. Numerous studies point out that ambient noise, often caused by traffic, can cause poor sleep and long-term health issues. In one study on women's bedroom environment, about 50% of participants found improved sleep quality as noise and light decreased.

Consider reducing the ambient noise, glare, and artificial lighting from gadgets such as alarm clocks to improve your bedroom environment. Make sure your bedroom is a quiet place to relax, clean, and enjoy.

Set your bedroom temperature

Heat in the body and bedroom can also have a profound impact on sleep quality.As you may have heard in the summer or in hot places, when it is too warm it can be very difficult to get a good night's sleep.One study found that the bedroom temperature affected sleep quality more than external noise Other studies reveal that increased body and bedroom temperatures can reduce the quality of sleep and increase awake time. For most people, about 70 ° F (20 ° C) seems to be a good temperature, although this depends on your tastes and behaviors.

Try to sleep and wake at consistent times

The circadian rhythm of your body functions on a set loop, and aligns with sunrise and sunset.It can help long-term sleep quality, being consistent with your sleep and waking times.One study noted poor sleep reported by participants who had irregular sleep patterns and went to bed late on the weekends.Other studies have pointed out that irregular sleep patterns can change your circadian rhythm and melatonin levels, which signal your brain to sleep.If you are dealing with sleep, try to get into the habit of waking up and going to bed at similar times. You may not even need an alarm after some weeks.

Relax and clear your mind in the evening

In the evening, many people have a pre-sleep routine to help them relax.Relaxation techniques have been shown to improve the quality of sleep and are another common method of treating insomnia. In one study in people who were ill, a relaxing massage improved sleep quality. Strategies include listening to relaxing music, reading a book, taking a hot bath, meditating, deep breathing ,and visualizing.

Try various methods, and find out what works best for you.

CONGRATS! YOU'VE DONE IT!

You've spent your time training and preparing yourself with the fewest possible tears to teach your child safely to sleep. I would like to extend my sincere thanks for trusting me and following my advice, and to remind you once again that all you need is time, patience, commitment, and faith to be successful.

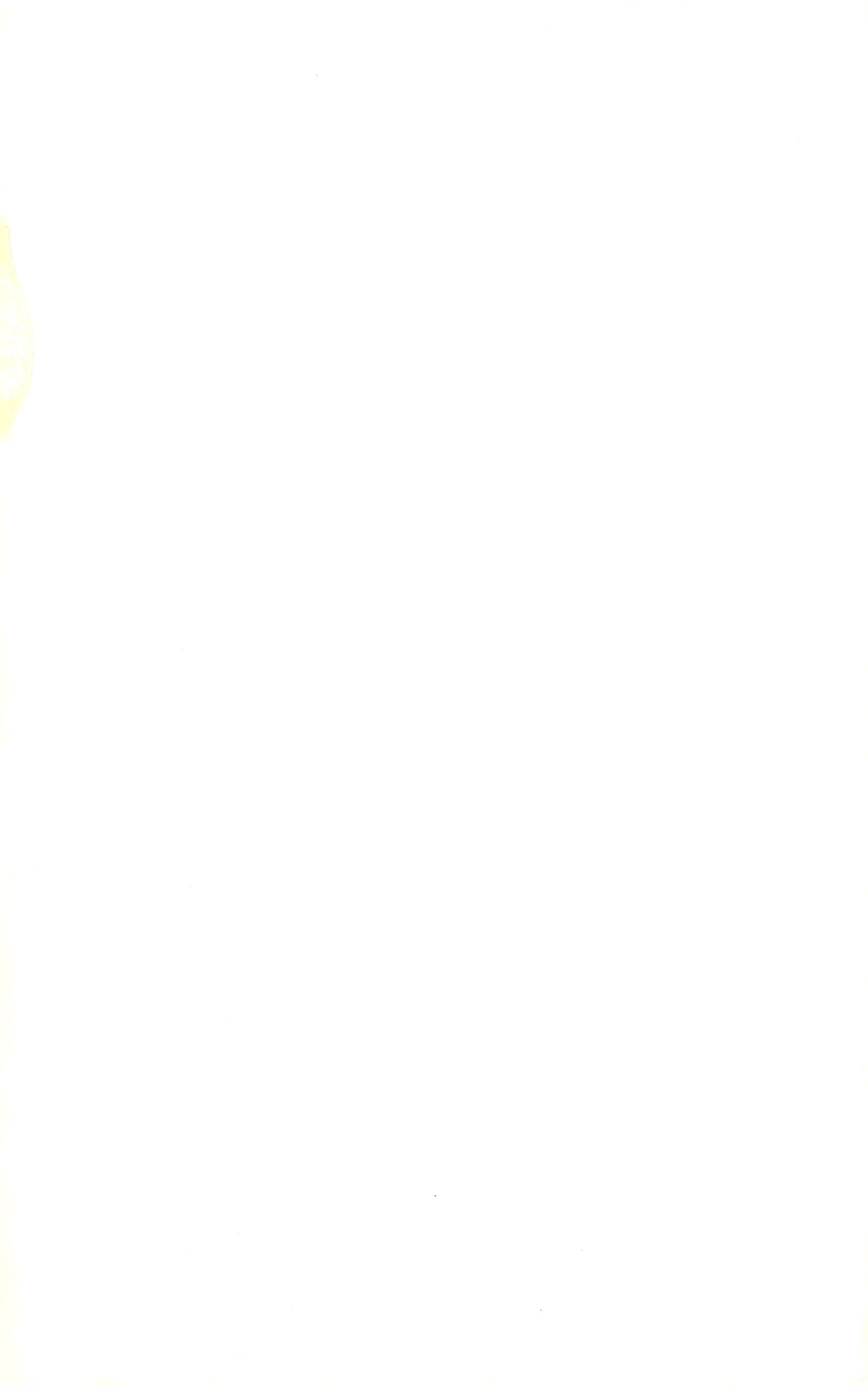